# A NEW HISTORY OF CATARACT SURGERY

# PART 1

# ANCIENT AND MEDIEVAL CATARACT COUCHING ALONG THE SILK ROAD

edited by
Christopher T. Leffler

ISBN: 978-90-6299-476-2

Wayenborgh Publishing
P.O. Box 20538
1001 NM Amsterdam, The Netherlands
www.historyophthalmology.com



Wayenborgh Publishing is an imprint of Kugler Publications, P.O. 20538, 1001 NM, Amsterdam, The Netherlands

# Table of Contents

## Chapter 2: The Ophthalmology of the Hellenistic Surgeon Antyllus . . . 115

*Matthias Witt*

# 1. Ancient and Medieval Cataract Couching along the Mediterranean and the Silk Road

Christopher T. Leffler, MD, MPH[1]

## Before Cataract Surgery

Over the millennia of human history, most societies have not performed cataract surgery. But they still practiced ophthalmology. Although the word *surgery* is derived etymologically from the word for hand, the first surgical tool was probably the mouth. Indigenous peoples of the Americas, who did not perform cataract couching, as far as anyone knows, still used the mouth as a healing tool, to suck, lick, or blow on the eye. Precouching societies also rubbed the eye to make it bleed to deal with ocular inflammation, corneal scars, and other conditions. Some societies operated on pterygia or superficial ocular growths by passing a thorn or hook below the opacity, lifting, and then, in some cases, cutting the opacity.[2]

Precouching societies also categorized eye diseases based on the degree and extent of pupillary color or brightening.[3] Of course, the pupil of the eye should look dark, and almost any disorder that produces a lighter pupil or cornea will scatter light and reduce vision.

## Late Bronze Age (2700 BCE)

Some scholars have seen hints that cataract surgery might have taken place during the Bronze Age, but none of the evidence is definitive. In Egypt, copper needles or probes were found in 1900 in the tomb of King Khasekhemwy at Abydos (ca. 2700 BCE).[4] Likewise, near the Saqqara pyramids close to Cairo, the tomb of Skar, one of the chief physicians in the fifth dynasty (ca. 2200 BCE) was found in 2001 to include several bronze surgical needles.[5] Because rods or probes can be used for the application of kohl or ointment, removal of foreign bodies, scraping the eye, nonophthalmic uses, and even nonmedical uses, the significance of these rods is unknown. In Egypt in the Old Kingdom, seven ophthalmic specialists are known. This total constitutes one-third of all known specialists.[6] The Ebers papyrus, the

---

1 Dept. of Ophthalmology, Virginia Commonwealth University, Richmond, Virginia.

2 Leffler et al. 2017.

3 Leffler et al. 2017; Leffler, Schwartz, Hadi, et al. 2015.

4 Ascaso 2009.

5 Ascaso 2009.

6 Blomstedt 2014.

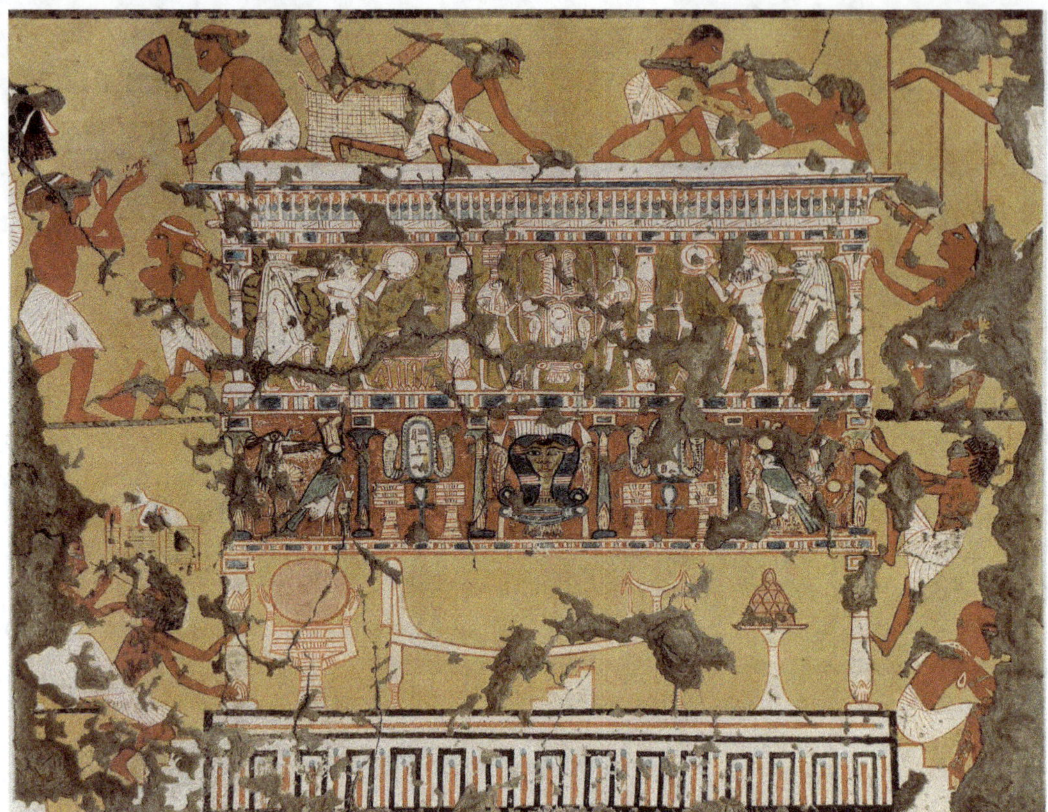

**Fig. 1.** The Tomb of Ipwy (c. 1200 BCE) at Thebes, Egypt. A doctor uses a rod to treat a workman's eye (lower left corner) (DeGaris Davies 1927).

Edwin-Smith papyrus, and other medical papyri of the period speak of medical recipes for ophthalmic conditions, but none refers to cataract surgery.[7]

A scene from the Tomb of Ipwy (ca. 1200 BCE) shows a worker at a construction site continuing to work while someone (possibly a doctor) approaches his eye with a rod (Fig. 1).[8] As someone above the worker is chiseling, it is possible that the doctor is trying to remove an ocular foreign body that had fallen into the eye.[9] The apparent repositioning of a dislocated shoulder in the upper right portion of the image is consistent with the idea that the figure depicts occupational injuries. Others have suggested the application of eye ointment or paint (kohl).[10]

---

7 Blomstedt 2014.

8 DeGaris Davies 1927. Plate XXXVII. Tomb of Apy (or Ipuy). North Wall, Lower part. Blomstedt 2014; Grzybowski, Ascaso 2014.

9 Blomstedt 2014.

10 DeGaris Davies 1927, p. 69.

None of the mummies that have been studied have any surgical incisions.[11] We have some stories about the personal lives of the royal families but are not told of any cataract surgeries.

In Babylon, the code of Hammurabi (reign 1792-1750 BCE) specified the charges and penalties for making an incision that heals a man's eye:

> If a physician [*asû*]...opened a man's temple with a bronze scalpel and healed the man's eye, he shall charge 10 shekels of silver (as his fee)... If an *asû*-physician has... opened a man's temple with a bronze scalpel and blinded the man's eye, they shall cut off his hand... If he opened his (the commoner's slave's) temple with a bronze scalpel and blinded his eye, he shall weigh out silver equal to half his value.[12]

The translator noted that although many have claimed that the code describes cataract surgery, in fact, "the procedure described cannot be verified by evidence from the medical corpus itself."[13] As translated, the procedure sounds like phlebotomy of a temporal blood vessel.

# The Book of Isaiah and Cyrus the Great (6th Century BCE)

Although the prophet Isaiah lived in the 8th century BCE, the work describing his prophecies underwent multiple revisions during the Jewish captivity in Babylon in the 6th century. That period of captivity ended after the Persian ruler Cyrus the Great captured Babylon. In fact, Cyrus the Great is compared to the Messiah in the book of Isaiah, and some scholars believe that in this book, Cyrus is the primary model for the Messiah who could liberate the Jewish people.[14]

The book of Isaiah is important from an ophthalmic perspective. Earlier Jewish works stated that God was responsible for creating people, including whether they could see. For instance, in Exodus 4:11, the Lord says, "Who gave man his mouth? Who makes him deaf or mute? Who gives him sight or makes him blind? Is it not I, the Lord?"

However, passages that correspond with the captivity in Babylon have for the first time statements that the deliverance of the people would be associated with cures of blindness, deafness, and lameness. For instance, Isaiah 29:18 records: "And in that day shall the deaf hear the words of the book, and the eyes of the blind shall see out of obscurity, and out of darkness." Isaiah 42:7 records: "To open the blind eyes, to bring out the prisoners from the prison, and them that sit in darkness out

---

11 Blomstedt 2014.

12 Geller 2010, p. 58.

13 Geller 2010, p. 184.

14 Isaiah 44:28, 45:1. Fried 2002.

of the prison house." This verse shows that "YHWH has obligated Cyrus to bring light into the present darkness, that is…to create the physical and political basis on which the peoples can live their own lives in peace and freedom."[15]

Similar passages are found in the Psalms. For instance, Psalm 146:8 records: "YHWH frees those who are in fetters, YHWH gives light to the blind; YHWH lifts up those who are bowed down."[16] The concepts in Psalm 146 are known to overlap substantially with the book of Isaiah: "The correlation to the book of Isaiah gives the psalm a multilayered dimension: YHWH's royal rule has been demonstrated… in the liberation of Israel (or the exiles) from political enslavement by the Babylonian world empire…"[17]

As it happens, Cyrus the Great asked the ruler of Egypt for his finest oculist (eye doctor).[18] And so we have the curious coincidence that the ruler who imported an eye doctor to Babylon is compared in the book of Isaiah with a Messiah who can cure blindness. It is interesting that Cyrus turned to Egypt for an eye doctor, instead of Taxila, in India. Taxila ultimately came under the rule of Cyrus and subsequent Persian kings.[19]

The postscript is that by one account, this oculist was indirectly responsible for the expansion of the Persian Empire to incorporate Egypt, reputed by the Greeks to be the site where cataract surgery originated.[20] The oculist requested by Cyrus was distraught about being uprooted from his family in Egypt. Therefore, he told Cambyses, the son and successor of Cyrus, to ask the Egyptian leader to send his daughter to be Cambyses' wife. The Egyptian leader instead sent the daughter of his defeated predecessor. When Cambyses discovered the ruse, he exacted vengeance by conquering Egypt in 525 BCE.[21]

# The Temple of Asclepius (350 BCE)

In ancient Greece, the Temple of Asclepius was the site of a number of ophthalmic healings, which might date to as early as the 4th century BCE. In the sanctuary of

---

15 Hossfeld et al. 2011, p. 615. Some hold that this verse actually relates to the Persian king Darius, even though Cyrus is explicitly mentioned elsewhere in Isaiah. Additionally, in the book of Isaiah (35:5-6), we find the passage: "Then the eyes of the blind shall be opened, and the ears of the deaf shall be unstopped. Then shall the lame man leap as an hart, and the tongue of the dumb sing: for in the wilderness shall waters break out, and streams in the desert." Karl Elliger is the historian who interpreted Isaiah 42:7.

16 Hossfeld et al. 2011, p. 608.

17 Hossfeld et al. 2011, pp. 610-611. This particular verse is held to correlate with Isaiah 42:7 (Hossfeld et al. 2011, p. 615)

18 Leffler, Klebanov, et al. 2020.

19 Naqvi 2003.

20 Leffler, Klebanov, et al. 2020.

21 Lang 1972; Beckwith 2015, p. 8; McEvilley 2002, p. 6.

Asclepius at Epidaurus, a stele was found, which was dated by the historian Cotter to about 350 BCE, and reads:

> Ambrosia from Athens, blind of one eye. She came as a supplicant to the god. As she walked about in the Temple she laughed at some of the cures as incredible and impossible, that the lame and the blind should be healed by merely seeing a dream. In her sleep she had a vision. It seemed to her that the god stood by her and said that he would cure her, but that in payment he would ask her to dedicate to the Temple a silver pig as a memorial of her ignorance. After saying this, he cut the diseased eyeball and poured in some drug. When day came she walked out sound.[22]

Another inscription from this stele at Epidaurus dated to 350 BCE reads:

> A man came as a supplicant to the god. He was so blind that of one of his eyes he had only the eyelids left—within them was nothing, but they were entirely empty. Some of those in the Temple laughed at his silliness to think that he could recover his sight when one of his eyes had not even a trace of the ball, but only the socket. As he slept a vision appeared to him. It seemed to him that the god prepared some drug, then, opening his eyelids, poured it into them. When day came he departed with the sight of both eyes restored.[23]

Another inscription from Epidaurus in 350 BCE reads:

> Alcetas of Halieis. The blind man saw a dream. It seemed to him that the god came up to him and with his fingers opened his eyes, and that he first saw the trees in the sanctuary. At daybreak he walked out sound.[24]

A final inscription from Epidaurus of 350 BCE reads:

> Hermon of Thasus. His blindness was cured by Asclepius. But, since afterwards he did not bring the thank-offerings, the god made him blind again. When he came back and slept again in the Temple, he [sc. the god] made him well.[25]

According to Sextus Empiricus, Asclepius was struck by lightning. A variety of explanations for the cause of the lightning strike were handed down by various historians from about 600 BCE onward.[26] None of these explanations had anything to do with ophthalmic healing, until the 3rd century BCE, when Phylarchus wrote that Asclepius was struck by lightning because he had restored the sight to the blinded sons of Phineus, as a favor to their mother Cleopatra, daughter of Erechtheus.[27] This

---

22  Inscriptiones Graecae 4.1.121-122: Stele 1.4; Cotter 1999, p. 17; Hamilton 1906, pp. 13-18.

23  Inscriptiones Graecae 4.1.121-122: Stele 1.9; Cotter 1999, p. 17.

24  Inscriptiones Graecae 4.1.121-122: Stele 1.18; Cotter 1999, p. 18.

25  Inscriptiones Graecae 4.1.121-122: Stele 2.22; Cotter 1999, p. 18.

26  Cotter 1999, p. 29.

27  Cotter 1999, p. 29.

timing corresponds with when Herophilus and Chrysippus of Cnidus were writing about ophthalmic anatomy and healing.

One ophthalmic healer, teacher, and miracle-worker connected with the Temple of Asclepius was Apollonius of Tyana (3 BCE-97 CE), whose life is understood from an early 3rd century account.[28] At the age of 14 years, Apollonius studied with a teacher from Phoenicia, which corresponds with present-day Lebanon.[29] Apollonius and his teacher settled at the Temple of Asclepius at Aegae, where he studied several philosophers: Plato and Chrysippus.[30] Plato (d. 347 BCE) wrote *Timaeus*, which discussed his theory of vision. Plato was stated by the medieval author Usaybia to have left behind children and family specializing in six areas of medicine, including Sergius, who specialized in ophthalmology.[31] There was a physician named Chrysippus of Cnidus of the 3rd century BCE who wrote an ophthalmic treatise.[32] However, in the context of philosophy, Apollonius' biographer must be referring to Chrysippus of Soli, also of the 3rd century BCE. This more prominent Chrysippus wrote about how vision takes place and also referred to restoration of vision through paracentesis, that is, cataract couching.[33]

At age 16, Apollonius left his teacher in order to better emulate Pythagoras. Apollonius became a vegetarian, went barefoot, and grew his hair long.[34] He recommended that treatment begin by providing laxatives.[35]

While he lived at the Temple at Aegae, he witnessed the cures brought about by Asclepius.[36] A rich patient from Cilicia surprised everyone at the temple by providing lavish offerings to the gods without first making a prayer request. Soon, the man was "supplicating the god [Asclepius] to restore to him one of his eyes that has fallen out."[37] Apollonius surmised that the patient had a guilty conscience, which Asclepius confirmed by appearing in the dream of a temple priest, saying that the patient "deserves to lose the other eye as well."[38] The priest investigated and learned that the patient had been seduced and was living in open sin with his stepdaughter. When the wife "surprised the two in bed, [she] had put out both her [the daughter's] eyes and one of his by stabbing them with her brooch-pin."

---

28 Philostratus, Conybeare 1912.

29 Philostratus, Conybeare 1912, p. 17.

30 Philostratus, Conybeare 1912, p. 17.

31 Usaybia 1971, p. 48. The other areas were diagnostics, dietetics, phlebotomy and cauterization, treatment of wounds, and setting broken bones. No surviving ancient source confirms this medieval idea that Plato had an ophthalmic disciple.

32 Leffler, Klebanov, et al. 2020.

33 Leffler, Klebanov, et al. 2020.

34 Philostratus, Conybeare 1912, p. 21.

35 Philostratus, Conybeare 1912, p. 20.

36 Philostratus, Conybeare 1912, p. 21.

37 Philostratus, Conybeare 1912, p. 25.

38 Philostratus, Conybeare 1912, p. 25.

This anecdote confirms that Apollonius was associated with the tradition of ophthalmic healing of the Asclepian temples.[39]

Apollonius traveled widely: to Scythia, around Asia Minor in silence, and as a sailor on the Mediterranean.[40] Apollonius is also connected with ophthalmic healings at the Temple of Serapis in Egypt, and in India, where he visited Taxila. Apollonius' story is unlikely to be historically accurate but demonstrates that an ancient audience would find it plausible that a 1st-century ophthalmic healer connected with the Temples of Asclepius and Serapis would practice in India.

## The Philosophers and Hypochyma (206 BCE)

Close to the start of the Common Era, we have stronger evidence of cataract surgery along the Nile and Indus Rivers. Regions close to these rivers were connected politically first during the Persian Empire and later with the conquests of Alexander the Great. He established Alexandria at the Nile Delta in 332 BCE, proceeded close to the Indus River, and captured Taxila in 326 BCE,[41] before dying at age 33 in Babylon.

Shortly after Alexander brought both Egypt and Taxila into the Greek-speaking world, we do find evidence that the Greeks became aware of cataract surgery. The philosopher Chrysippus of Soli (c. 279-c. 206 BCE) mentioned couching of cataracts. Chrysippus' works have been lost, but he was cited by Simplicius of Cilicia (c. 490-c. 560), who, in reviewing the philosophy of Aristotle and Chrysippus, wrote:[42]

> For although blindness comes about from sight, [change] does not [occur] in the reverse direction as well. And because of this Chrysippus raised the question whether those suffering from a cataract [ὑποχυθέντας, *hypochythentas*] but able to recover sight after a couching of the eye [ἐκπαρακεντήσεως, *ekparakenteseos*] should be called blind, and [he raised the same question] in the case of those whose eyelids are [naturally] shut: for since the capacity [to see] exists, they resemble someone [voluntarily] keeping his eyes shut, or someone prevented by a screen [παραπέτασμα, *parapetasma*] from seeing, since if this [screen] is removed [ἀφαιρεθέντος, *aphairethentos*] he is in no way prevented from seeing. So it is not from privation to possession that such a change comes about. But [Aristotle] is here considering the kind of privation which consists in a disability. For from such a [privation] there is no return to the [corresponding] possession.[43]

---

39  Philostratus, Conybeare 1912, pp. 29, 33. This healing occurred before Apollonius was 20 years old.

40  Philostratus, Conybeare 1912, pp. x, 35, 37; Priaulx 1860.

41  Naqvi 2003.

42  Simplicius, Kalbfleisch 1907, p. 401.

43  Simplicius, Gaskin 2013, p. 143.

As Chrysippus' mention predates any established couching tools, or other mentions of the technique by centuries, we might wonder if Simplicius was simply using the language of his own day to paraphrase a more general statement by Chrysippus about healing the blind. However, the botanist Theophrastus (371-287 BCE) had used the term παρακεντοῦντες (*parakentountes*) in a nonmedical sense to describe "stirring it [a heap] with poles."[44] Moreover, multiple subsequent philosophers who cited Chrysippus also referred to this condition. Of the 2nd-century BCE philosopher Carneades, it was written that "his eyes went blind [ὑποχυθῆναι, *hypochythenai*]"—a form of the word almost identical to that attributed to Chrysippus.[45] Carneades apparently did not have surgery to restore his vision. Philosopher Maximus of Tyre in the 2nd century CE wrote: "When medical science comes to the rescue...to remove the blockage so as to uncover it and restore its outward passage....The misfortune of physical embodiment covers it over with a thick mist [ὑποκεχύσθαι, *hypokethysthai*], which confounds its powers of vision..."[46] Theophilus of Antioch in the 2nd century CE referred to "cataracts [ὑποκεχυμένους, *hypokechymenous*] over the eyes of your soul" and how God will "couch [παρακεντήσει, *parakentesei*] the eyes of your soul."[47] Medical authors well before Simplicius had begun using forms such as *hypochyma*.[48] Therefore, Simplicius was not using a language restricted to his own day—he was using the language of philosophers since Chrysippus and Carneades. Thus, we believe that cataract surgery was known in the Greek-speaking world at the time of Chrysippus of Soli.

The term used by Chrysippus of Soli, *hypochyma*, continued to be used in ophthalmic works, many of which discussed cataract surgery. In the 1st century CE, an anonymous papyrus from Egypt entitled *Traité Sur L'Enseignement de la Chirurgie* contains a fragment of the surgeon Archibios. The work mentions Hippocrates' teaching (Life is short and the art is long) and then states that it is absurd that students would not know the definitions of cataract (ὑπόχυμα, *hypochyma*), hydrops (ὕδρωφ), and the rudiments of surgery.[49]

An Egyptian papyrus from the 2nd century AD (*Questionnaire d'Ophthalmologie*) reviews the differences between glaucoma (γλαύχωα), cataract (ὑπόχυμα, *hypochyma*), staphyloma, and pterygium (πτερύγιον, *pterygion*).[50] Glaucoma could not be treated. Cataract implied a white color in the pupil and was more treatable than glaucoma, though cataract surgery was not explicitly specified. Pterygium was operated with a hook and staphyloma with a needle, while a flux of humors was cauterized.[51]

---

44 Theophrastus, Hort 1916, vol. I, pp. 470-471.

45 Diogenes, Hicks 1925, pp. 440-443.

46 Maximus of Tyre, Trapp 1997, p. 87.

47 Theophilus of Antioch, Grant 1970, pp. 4-11.

48 Leffler, Schwartz, 2020a, pp. 1-46; Leffler et al. 2017; Leffler, Schwartz, Hadi, et al. 2015.

49 Marganne 1981, pp. 7-8. The papyrus is denoted BKT 3.22-26, inv. 9764 = Pack2 2354.

50 Marganne 1981, pp. 266-267. The papyrus is denoted P. Ross. Georg. 1. 20; Pack2 2343.

51 Marganne 1994, pp. 120-121.

Of note, the Greeks did not claim the discovery of cataract surgery for themselves. The author called pseudo-Galen, because he lived close in time to Galen of Pergamon (c. 129-199 CE), was apparently familiar with the practice of medicine in Egypt.[52] Pseudo-Galen in *Introductio Sive Medicus* contrasted the Greek way of learning medicine from the Gods with the Egyptian emphasis on empiric observation:[53]

> But the Egyptians also used plants and other remedies, as Homer attests when he says: 'the Egyptian, where the fertile earth produces many different drugs, many being beneficial when mixed, many being harmful'. Moreover, it is from the dissection of dead bodies when they are embalmed that many treatments used in surgery came to be discovered by the first doctors; others, it is said, were discovered by chance, such as paracentesis [παρακεντεῖν, *parakentein*] of the eyes of patients suffering from cataracts [ὑποκεχυμένους, *hypokechymenous*], thanks to the encounter of a goat which, afflicted from cataracts [ὑποχυθεῖσα, *hypochytheisa*], recovered its sight after a sharp rush leaf became stuck in its eye. It is also said that the enema was invented by watching the ibis, which fills its neck with Nile water or sea water, like an enema syringe, and injects itself below with its beak...[54]

It may enhance the credibility of pseudo-Galen to learn that the enema was indeed described in Egypt as early as the Ebers papyrus of 1500 BCE.[55]

In Ptolemaic Alexandria, the major surgeons and anatomists were Herophilus and Erasistratus. The teacher of Erasistratus was Chrysippus of Cnidus, who was active from about 320 to 280 BCE, wrote the now-lost *Treatments for Sight* and studied under Aethlius (and perhaps the doctors in his family).[56] The works of Chrysippus of Cnidus survived at least to the time of Galen.[57] The doctors in the Chrysippus family had connections to Egypt.[58] In the early Common Era, Demosthenes Philalethes wrote a lost treatise of ophthalmology.

# Herophilus of Alexandria (280 BCE)

Having established that the Greeks were aware of cataract couching shortly after Alexander the Great expanded the Greek world, we might now make the case that

---

52  Jouanna, Allies 2012, p. 15.

53  Galien, Kuhn 1827, vol. 14, p. 675. *Introductio Sive Medicus* (Kühn 14.674-797) contains the relevant passage (Kühn 14.674-676).

54  Jouanna, Allies 2012, pp. 15-16.

55  Friedenwald, Morrison 1940.

56  Berrey 2014.

57  Berrey 2014.

58  Chrysippus' grandfather, also of Cnidus, studied medicine under Philistion of Sicily but had travelled to Egypt with the astronomer Eudoxus (Berrey 2014). Another Chrysippus, the son of the Chrysippus who taught Erasistratus, was the doctor to Ptolemy Philadelphpus in 279 BCE (Berrey 2014).

one particular surgeon was aware of the procedure. Herophilus of Alexandria was primarily known as an anatomist and surgeon. Our knowledge of the surgical practices of the Alexandrian Herophilus is limited. He alluded to the extraction of a tooth and discussed obstetric complications.[59] Indeed, according to Tertullian, Herophilus had a surgical instrument to produce abortions ("fetus slayer"), which had already been possessed by Hippocrates.[60]

Herophilus and Erasistratus were reputed to have performed anatomic dissections on condemned criminals while they were still alive. Some have questioned the veracity of these accounts, but the historian von Staden argues for their plausibility.

Herophilus once treated a philosopher named Diodorus Cronus, who had a dislocated shoulder. This philosopher had previously argued that motion was paradoxical. Herophilus told his patient that the shoulder could not have moved, because the philosopher had already proved that motion was impossible. Herophilus stated: "Your shoulder was dislocated either being in the place where it was or being where it was not; but [it was dislocated] neither where it was nor where it was not; therefore it has not been dislocated." The suffering sophist then begged Herophilus to treat him by the precepts of medicine rather than philosophy.[61]

A circumstantial case can be made that Herophilus was familiar with cataract couching. He wrote a now-lost treatise *On Eyes*, dissected the eyes of humans, and is credited by von Staden with the discovery of the optic nerve.[62] Herophilus compared the retina to a net.[63]

Ophthalmic passages from the early works of Cornelius Celsus (c. 25 BC-50 AD) and Pliny the Elder referred to cataract surgery and also cited Herophilus and Erasistratus.

Herophilus is only mentioned one time in Galen's 345-page *On Diseases and Symptoms*. This occurrence is most directly with respect to Herophilus' understanding that the optic nerves carry sensory *pneuma* to the eye. However, the occurrence is also in the context of how contralateral pupillary dilation in response to unilateral eye closure is a positive prognostic indicator for cataract surgery.[64]

Other findings suggesting that Herophilus was familiar with cataract surgery are (1) the importance of posterior uveal roughness to the couching procedure and (2) the humoral understanding of cataract pathophysiology, both discussed later.

---

59  Von Staden 1989, p. 403.

60  Von Staden 1989, pp. 190-404.

61  Von Staden 1989, pp. 49-57.

62  Von Staden 1989, pp. 20-423.

63  Von Staden 1989, p. 205.

64  See chapter on pupillary responses.

# The Cornea (3rd Century BCE)

The word *cornea* is derived etymologically from the word for horn, and this comparison of a cornea to a horn probably dates from the era of Herophilus, because the comparison was made in the early anatomic passages of Celsus and Rufus, which cited Herophilus.[65] Of course, the cornea does not really look like a horn. But the earliest definitions of the cornea, in Celsus and Rufus, look at the combination of cornea and sclera as one contiguous structure, which happens to be thinner and transparent in the front. Perhaps, the white sclera does look a bit more like a horn. Galen in the 2nd century distinguished the sclera from the cornea as anatomic structures, as we do today. Galen was able to convince himself that the cornea does resemble a horn if the horn is sliced so thin that it becomes transparent.

# The Posterior Uveal Surface (3rd Century BCE)

Herophilus taught that the posterior surface of the uvea was rough. As Rufus of Ephesus wrote:

> The perforated body [the iris] is smooth on the outside where it meets with the horn-like coat [the cornea], but rough on the side that is turned away, as Herophilus says, resembling the skin of a grape, being interwoven with blood-vessels. This coat is called the 'second' on account of its position, 'perforated on the basis of its structure, 'grape-like' on the basis of its resemblance, and 'chorioid' on the ground that it is interlaced with blood-vessels like the foetal membrane (chorion).[66]

We might note in passing that the comparison of the uvea to a grape was not found in Hippocratic medicine. The ancient Babylonians did compare it to a grape over a millennium earlier, but a continuity of the teachings cannot be established. Authors who cited Herophilus, such as Celsus or Galen, also compared the uvea to a grape or raisin.[67] The comparison of the eye's choroid with the chorion, the outermost layer of the placenta, is consistent with Herophilus' specialty of obstetrics.

Herophilus' teaching that the posterior uveal surface is rough actually associates his work with cataract couching. It might seem somewhat odd that the teaching of the rough posterior uveal surface has survived for millennia. Galen simply stated that the soft inner uveal surface protected the crystalline lens (in *De Usu Partium*). However, in many works, the inner uveal surface was believed to be quite important with respect to cataract couching for two reasons. First, the couching needle had to be sharp enough to penetrate the sclera, but if the needle was too sharp, it would tear the iris. The danger of uveal trauma during cataract couching because of the

---

65  Von Staden 1989, pp. 205-206.

66  Von Staden 1989, p. 205.

67  Gordon 1933.

roughnesses on its posterior surface was emphasized by subsequent authors. Second, the roughnesses on the posterior surface of the uvea or ciliary body were believed to be helpful in retaining the couched cataract in the vitreous.

The surgeon Antyllus (2nd to 4th centuries), possibly of Alexandria, wrote that the "viscosity" of the uvea helped it avoid perforation by the cataract needle.[68] Likewise, Hunain of 9th-century Baghdad recorded:

> The grape-like tunic (uvea, iris)…is rich in veins to nourish the cornea, and it is (moreover) soft in order that it may not injure the lens by its friction; therefore it is furnished on the inside with tufts (villi) from which is suspended the cataract, when we operate on it. But it is smooth on the outside in order that it may not be hurt by the cornea.[69]

Hunain's cataract couching method specified:

> After you have pierced it (the eye), beware of turning your needle in the wrong direction and of reaching the back of the uvea from inside and tearing it, for that would destroy its pupil and it is (an injury) not likely to be cured.[70]

Ibn Isa, of 11th-century Baghdad, drew much of his cataract couching method from Antyllus. Ibn Isa recorded that the posterior uveal anatomy was evident when operating for cataract:

> The uveal covering lies in front of the vitreous…Its [the uvea's] inner aspect presents a tufted appearance that serves two purposes, one of which is to hold in place the semi-fluid vitreous. One notices in it, when operating on a cataract, an impression of irregularities.[71]

In his cataract method, Ibn Isa noted:

> The uveal tunic is smooth and covered with moisture; when the needle touches it, it glides over and away from it. Moreover, the point of the instrument (*miḥyaṭ*) is purposely made round so that it will not cut or wound the uveal tissues, although it is true that if it were very sharp at the anterior end its introduction would be easier for the operator.[72]

---

68 Antyllus wrote, according to Rhazes' *Continens*: "The uvea [*'inabî*] is easily repelled, without being perforated, by the instrument, because it recedes because of its viscosity [*viscositatem, luzūǧa*] and because the tip of the needle is not very sharp." (Meyerhof 1932). In this case, the uveal tissue in question is the ciliary body. According to Oliver Kahl (personal communication, 2021), the term translated as "viscosity" reads in the Arabic *luzūǧa*; this word covers the semantic range of "viscidity, stickiness, glueyness" as well as "elasticity".

69 Hunain, Meyerhof 1928 pp. 9-10.

70 Hunain, Meyerhof 1928, p. 122.

71 Ibn Isa, Wood 1936, p. 18.

72 Ibn Isa, Wood 1936, p. 178.

Ibn Isa instructed that during cataract couching, after penetration of the needle:

> Now turn the needle until you see its point above the cataract, as this will be visible through the transparent cornea; also during the act of rotating the head of the needle you will be able to see the uvea and recognize its hairy processes (villi). You will now understand the reason why the point of the needle should not be too sharp; if it were it might wound the uveal tunic during these manipulations.[73]

Ibn Isa compared the expansion of the pupil during cataract couching to childbirth:

> Anyone may ask how…can the cataract be attached to the processes of the uveal covering? I reply that when the needle is passed between the two tunics it comes in contact with both the cataract and the uvea and at the same time the operator causes an enlargement of the pupil, just as in childbirth the elastic uterus, after expanding to allow the passage of the child, once more returns to its normal condition. In the same way the ocular tunics and the dilated pupil resume their usual state after cessation of the pressure put upon them by the cataract operation.[74]

Given that neither Ibn Isa nor his source Antyllus was known for obstetrics, one might wonder if the original source was the obstetrician Herophilus.

The uveal surface was also believed to hold the cataract in the vitreous. According to Ibn Isa,

> Occasionally the usual velvety surface of the ciliary body is found to have become slippery and does not keep back the cataract.[75]

Ammar of Cairo understood the uveal tissues to adhere to the cataract:

> Once you see that the cataract is luxated posteriorly and the pupil has become clear with the cataract having reached the ciliary body processes, keep the needle firmly in place [stationary] for some time, until the process situated on the inner surface of the ciliary body have taken hold of the cataract [by suction and adhesion]. Only then lift the needle off the cataract.[76]

# Phlegm and the Eye (3rd Century BCE)

The Greeks had numerous humoral theories of disease, although not all Greek doctors emphasized humoral causes. Herophilus subscribed to the humoral theory

---

73  Ibn Isa, Wood 1936, p. 185.
74  Ibn Isa, Wood 1936, p. 178.
75  Ibn Isa, Wood 1936, pp. 185-186.
76  Blodi et al. 1993, p. 154.

of disease, according to Galen.[77] The pseudo-Galen *Introductio sive medicus* (1st century) recorded:

> Some people attributed both the constitution of things that are in accordance with nature and the cause of things that are contrary to nature to the humours (Χυμοις, *chymois*) alone, as did Praxagoras and Herophilus.[78]

With respect to cataract, the early Greco-Roman works agreed with the Indian that there was some sort of pathologic humor (χυμός, *chymos*) that had settled in the eye to cause the disorder. Thus, as noted earlier, the Greeks eventually called the lesion treated by couching *hypochyma*, and the Romans called it *suffusio* (suffusion). It was not generally clear in the Greco-Roman system exactly what fluid was causing a couchable lesion—phlegm, bile, or blood. However, occasional Greek references *did* specify abnormal phlegm settling in the eye. The work *Diseases 2*, traditionally attributed to Hippocrates, referred to phlegm in the pupil of the eye, but the patient recovered without surgery:

> When the head becomes overheated...the phlegm in it melts...it goes partly to the nostrils, partly to the mouth...Patients see unclearly, in this condition, when phlegm enters the small vessels of their eyes; for the pupil becomes more watery and turbid, so that the clear part of the eye is no longer as clear as it was, and thus the image does not appear in it, when it wishes to see, the same as when it was clear and pure. This patient generally recovers in forty days.[79]

*Diseases 2* might be a composite work, with certain portions, including the above-mentioned quotation, postdating the Hippocratic era.[80] The corresponding passage from the older portion of *Diseases 2*, which is believed to date from the Hippocratic era, states that this disease ends if "fluid and mucus break out through his nostrils or ears," though "the sight is snatched from his eyes, and he seems to see only the half of faces."[81] Thus, the older version did not specify phlegm entering the eye.

A Greek ophthalmic papyrus (*Traité d'Ophtalmologie*) from the first half of the 3rd century BCE from Hibeh, Egypt, has been attributed, based on the style, to either Diocles of Carystus or Chrysippus of Cnidus; however, the fragmentary nature of the document makes attribution difficult. The treatise mentions *pneuma* (πνευμα), phlegm (φλέγμα), and hardness (σκληρότες, *sklerotes*) as relevant to ophthalmology, possibly with respect to mucoid discharge or mattering.[82]

---

77  Von Staden 1989, p. 243.

78  Von Staden 1989, p. 243.

79  Hippocrates, Potter 1988, pp. 170-171. (Littré VII 8)

80  Jouanna, Allies 2012, p. 236.

81  Hippocrates, Potter, 1988, p. 185. (Littré VII 20)

82  Marganne 1981, p. 46. Papyrus: Pack2 342.

In a Greek papyrus (*Traité d'Ophtalmologie*) of the 2nd century BCE from the Roman province of Arsinoë, Egypt, there is the suggestion of a pathologic phlegmatic, glassy humor in the eye, causing a coloration of the pupil described as *glaukomaton*:

> However, as the humors [ὑγρὼν, *hygron*] of the eye have been crushed and the wound is contused, this disorder typically produces a gray-blue coloration [γλαύκωσιν, *glaukosin*]. In effect, the gray-blue colorations [γλαυκωμάτων, *glaukomaton*] appear when a phlegmatic [φλεγματῶδες, *phlegmatodes*] humor [ὑγρόν, *hygron*] in the region of the pupil, and that engenders a cold: that is also why this humor is glassy [ὑαλῶδες, *hyalodes*] in color and consistence.[83]

Celsus noted that "wild poppy heads" could help to "check the flow of phlegm into the eyes."[84] In Celsus' work, the idea of phlegm in the eye is most strongly related to the Indian concepts, because phlegm accounted for *hypochysis*—the same term Celsus used for the couchable lesion:

> Cataract also, which the Greeks call *hypochysis*, sometimes interferes with the vision of the eye. When it has become long established it is to be treated surgically. In its earliest stages it may be dispersed occasionally by certain measures: it is useful to let blood from the forehead or nostrils, to cauterize the temporal blood vessels, to bring out phlegm by gargling, to inhale smoke, to anoint the eyes with acrid medicaments. That regimen is best which makes phlegm thin.[85]

Celsus' recommendations resemble those of Suśruta for *Adhimantha* (ophthalmia) caused by *kapha*.[86]

In his veterinary work, Vegetius of the late 4th century was explicit that cataracts that resembled mucus were suitable for couching.

The humoral basis for the various colors of cataract became most advanced in the works of Ṣalāḥ al-Dīn al-Kaḥḥāl of 13th-century Hama, Syria. Ṣalāḥ al-Dīn believed that excess mucous caused most cataracts, and he separated black and yellow bile, in the manner of the Greek authors.[87]

In the Ayurvedic literature, phlegm (*kapha*) was considered the only humor that produced an ophthalmic lesion suitable for couching. In the Chinese literature, there were some mentions of phlegm as a cause of eye illness. Treatise on the *Origins and Symptoms of Disease*, compiled by Chao Yuanfang (550-630) of China in 610 CE was the first to describe screens *zhang* and shades *yi* in the eye and attributed

---

83  Marganne 1981, p. 53. Papyrus: Pack2 2344.
84  Celsus, Spencer 1938, p. 62. Book V.
85  Celsus, Spencer 1938, p. 222. Book VI.
86  Sushruta, Bhishagratna 1916, vol. III, p. 41.
87  Blodi et al. 1993, p. 279.

these, and other eye conditions, to phlegm in the eye.[88] Yuanfang's treatise did not mention cataract surgery. A later medieval Japanese work, *Ishinpo*, presented in 984 CE, equated a phlegm-induced eye disease whose description he attributed to Yuangfang with a condition treated with the golden needle:

> When afflicted with cataract ['clear blindness'], the pupil of the eye does not actually show anything abnormal…the afflicted cannot see anything. If the Viscera are weak and afflicted with Wind Illness and if there is phlegm, one gets sick.[89]

In some later medieval Chinese works, the substance was not phlegm, but fat. Eye disease was attributed to wind arising from the liver, or "brain fluid flowing down" or *Nao liu* ("the brain fat flows down") to the eye.[90]

Later, *Essential Subtleties on the Silver Sea* again attributed a number of eye illnesses to phlegm or "phlegm and fluid" (*tan yin*), though it is not clear that the screens and shades treated with the golden needle were caused in this manner.[91]

## The *Book of Tobit* (200 BCE)

The *Book of Tobit* is set in the 8th century BCE but was written about 200 BCE in Aramaic and then translated into Hebrew.[92] Tobit, an elderly Jewish man living in Nineveh after being held captive in Assyria, became blind after he fell asleep outside in his garden and bird droppings (from sparrows in the Greek translation) fell into his eyes, producing a film.[93] The Aramaic term used to describe the white ocular film was *ḥwrwryn*, and this became leucoma in the Greek translation.[94] This injury has been interpreted as a divine punishment, or, alternatively, as a satire of the Mesopotamian physicians, who would use bird or bat excrement as an ophthalmic treatment. According to the Greek recension, the more his physicians treated his eye, the worse it became.[95] His son Tobias was instructed by the angel Raphael to capture a fish that jumped from the Tigris River and to extract the fish gall as an ophthalmic treatment for his father:

---

88 Kovacs, Unschuld 1998, pp. 30-32. Treatise name: *Zhubing yuan hou lun.*

89 Triplett 2019.

90 Deshpande, Fan 2012, "brain fluid" in Indian Classic of Discussion on Eyes, Tianzhu jing lunyan, p. 80; "brain fat" in Treatise of Bodhisattva Nagarjuna on eye (diseases), *Longshu pusa yanlun*, pp. 93, 109; "brain fat" in Nagarjuna's Comprehensive Treatise, *Longmu zong lun*, pp. 138, 146.

91 Kovacs, Unschuld 1998, pp. 126, 128, 193, 255, 257-258, 313, 393, 397, 407, 440, 451, 455, 457-459. Essential Subtleties on the Silver Sea, *Yin-hai jing-wei.*

92 Attia 2018.

93 Attia 2018.

94 Attia 2018.

95 Attia 2018.

> Then Raphael said to Tobias…'I know that his eyes will be opened. Sprinkle / scatter the gall of the fish and the medicine will make the white films contract and peel off from his eyes, and your father will look up and see the light.'[96]

When Tobias arrived at his father's house, the father ran outside, but stumbled, apparently just after exiting the door. Then, Tobias placed the fish gall on his father's eyes, and the vision was restored (Fig. 2):

> Now, the gall of the fish was in his hand, and he blew into his eyes and held him… Then he laid the medicine on him, and it worked. And he scaled it off with both hands from the corner of his eyes.[97]

Perhaps, the story of Tobit can teach us that in antiquity, blindness was sometimes treated within families, on advice from third parties, in an outdoor setting, with the patient lower than the doctor, by rubbing using both hands or blowing medicine on the eyes.

The type of fish was not specified in Tobit, but in Mesopotamian tradition, carp scales were used in magical rituals.[98] Carp gall was recommended as an electuary to be rubbed on the eyelids for cataract by Ibn Isa of 11th-century Baghdad.[99]

Carp gall was also recommended for the eyes in East Asia. The Indian Classic on Eye Diseases, attributed to a Buddhist monk named Xie from Long Shang at the Western border of the Tang Empire, recommended carp gallbladder (*Li yu dan*) taken orally for an eye with "red flesh due to wind-and-heat."[100]

The work *Ishinpo*, presented to the Japanese court in 984 CE, mentioned that the golden needle is used to treat a cataract ("blue-white shade"), which helps the patient see the sun as if the clouds had been opened. But in addition to this surgical treatment, *Ishinpo* recommended both oral and topically applied carp gall for the condition.[101]

The works of Antyllus, and derivative works, such as those of Ibn Isa, Ammar, Ṣalāḥ al-Dīn, and Ibn Sina (Avicenna), stated that eating fish would thicken a cataract and, therefore, generally promoted cataract development, but on the other hand, fish could be taken preoperatively to help the cataract mature.

---

96 Attia 2018. Tobit 11:7.

97 Attia 2018. Tobit 11:11.

98 Attia 2018.

99 Ibn Isa, Wood 1936, p. 182.

100 Deshpande, Fan 2012, p. 86. Treatise: *Tianzhu jing lunyan*.

101 Mishima 2004, pp. 56, 67, 68. Condition: *seimo* or *aikishihi*. Triplett 2019, pp. 89-90.

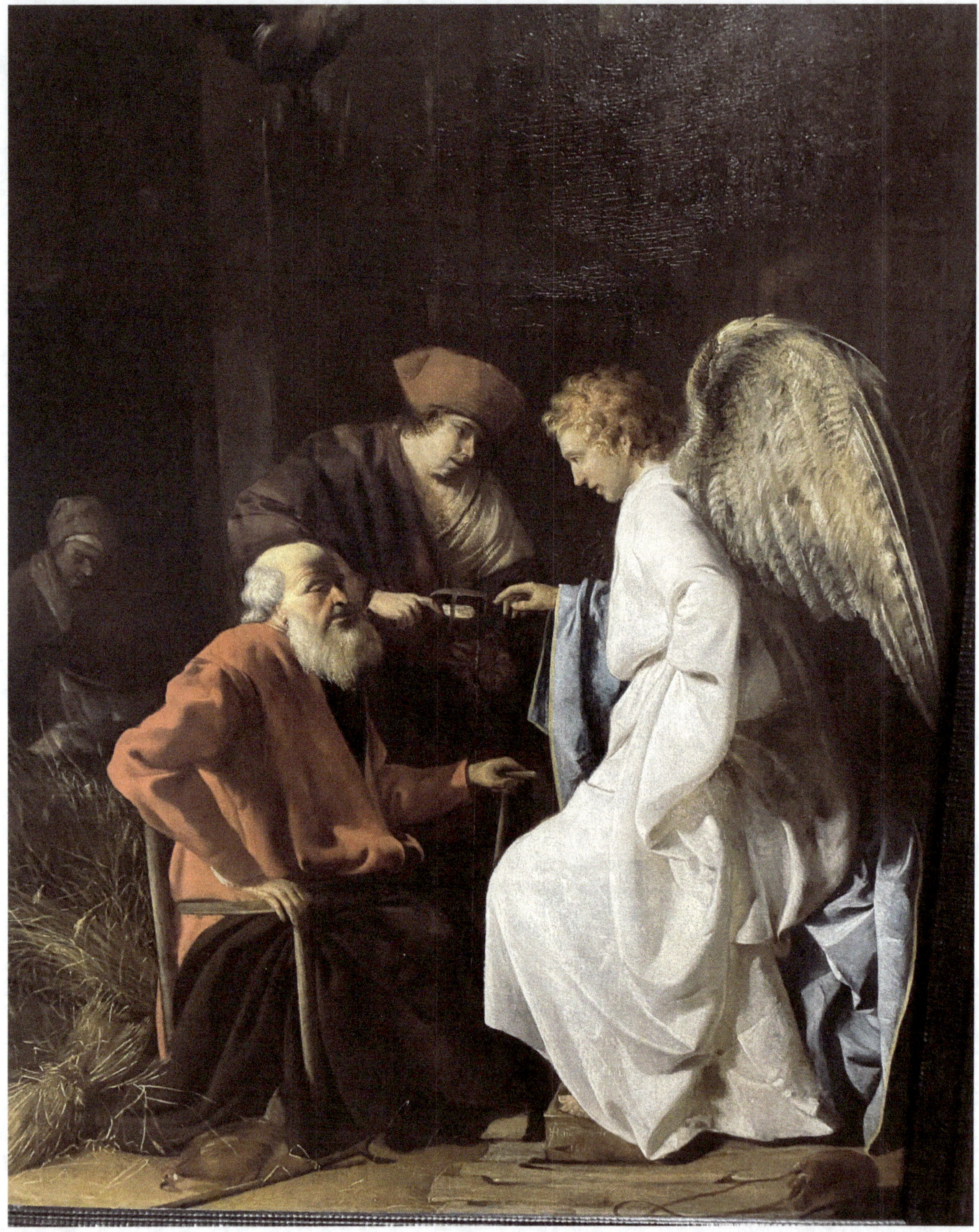

**Fig. 2.** *Tobias and the Angel Curing Tobit of Blindness*, painted by Dutch author Simon Henrixz. van Amersfoort in 1630.

## The Glassy Eye (2nd Century BCE)

Glass manufacture was advanced along the Mediterranean. Roman glass could be tinged green (most commonly), but sometimes amber or other colors, depending on impurities.[102] Glass played a role in the physiology and pathophysiology in the Greco-Roman works. Praxagoras of Cos, who taught Herophilus, had a complicated humoral theory, which included a glassy (vitreous) humor as one of the fundamental humors.[103] In a discussion of eye anatomy, which cited Herophilus, Rufus of Ephesus mentioned the vitreous (*hyaloeide*).[104] Today, we still call the clear fluid in the back of the eye the vitreous humor.

In the ancient Greek literature, a glassy appearance to the eye could also represent pathology. As noted earlier, a Greek papyrus from Egypt in the 2nd century BCE noted a pathologic glassy humor in the eye. Apsyrtos of Bithynia (fl. 3rd century CE) wrote: "When γλαύκωμα [glaucoma] occurs, lancing is useless because [the disease] is incurable. It is a result of a so-called glazing of the eye (ὑάλωμα, *hyaloma*, glassy disease) rather like a λευκη [*leuke*] pebble."[105] On the other hand, Aëtius of Amida, drawing on the work of Demosthenes Philalethes of the 1st century CE, noted a cataract appearing similar to glass (ὑελίζει, *hyelizei*, "bottle green"), which was not specified as untreatable.[106] This idea was promulgated by subsequent Arabic authors. Ṣalāḥ al-Dīn al-Kaḥḥāl of 13th-century Hama, Syria, wrote in *The Book of Light of the Eyes* that one type of cataract "has the color of glass."[107] Khalifah of 13th-century Aleppo described a cataract "the color of glass, also known under the name of pearly cataract. It approaches being suitable for surgery."[108]

In the Ayurvedic literature of India, the *Suśrutasaṃhitā* and the *Aṣṭāṅgahṛdayasaṃhitā* also described some diseased eyes as glassy but considered them unsuitable for surgery.

## The Glaucous Pupil (2nd Century BCE)

As noted earlier, ancient cultures described many blinding conditions by the color of the pupil. Historically, languages often make no distinction between blue, green, and gray, using the same term to describe all of these colors.[109] Many corneal conditions, such as scarring, band keratopathy, keratitis, vitamin A deficiency, or

---

102 Leffler, Schwartz, Hadi, et al. 2015.

103 Praxagoras, Steckerl 1958, pp. 73-75.

104 Von Staden 1989, p. 206; Shastid 1913, vol. 11, p. 8580.

105 Leffler, Schwartz, Hadi, et al. 2015.

106 Aëtius of Amida, Waugh 2000, pp. 85-86.

107 Blodi et al. 1993, p. 276.

108 Blodi et al. 1993, p. 213.

109 Leffler, Schwartz, Hadi, et al. 2015; Leffler, Schwartz, Giliberti, et al. 2015.

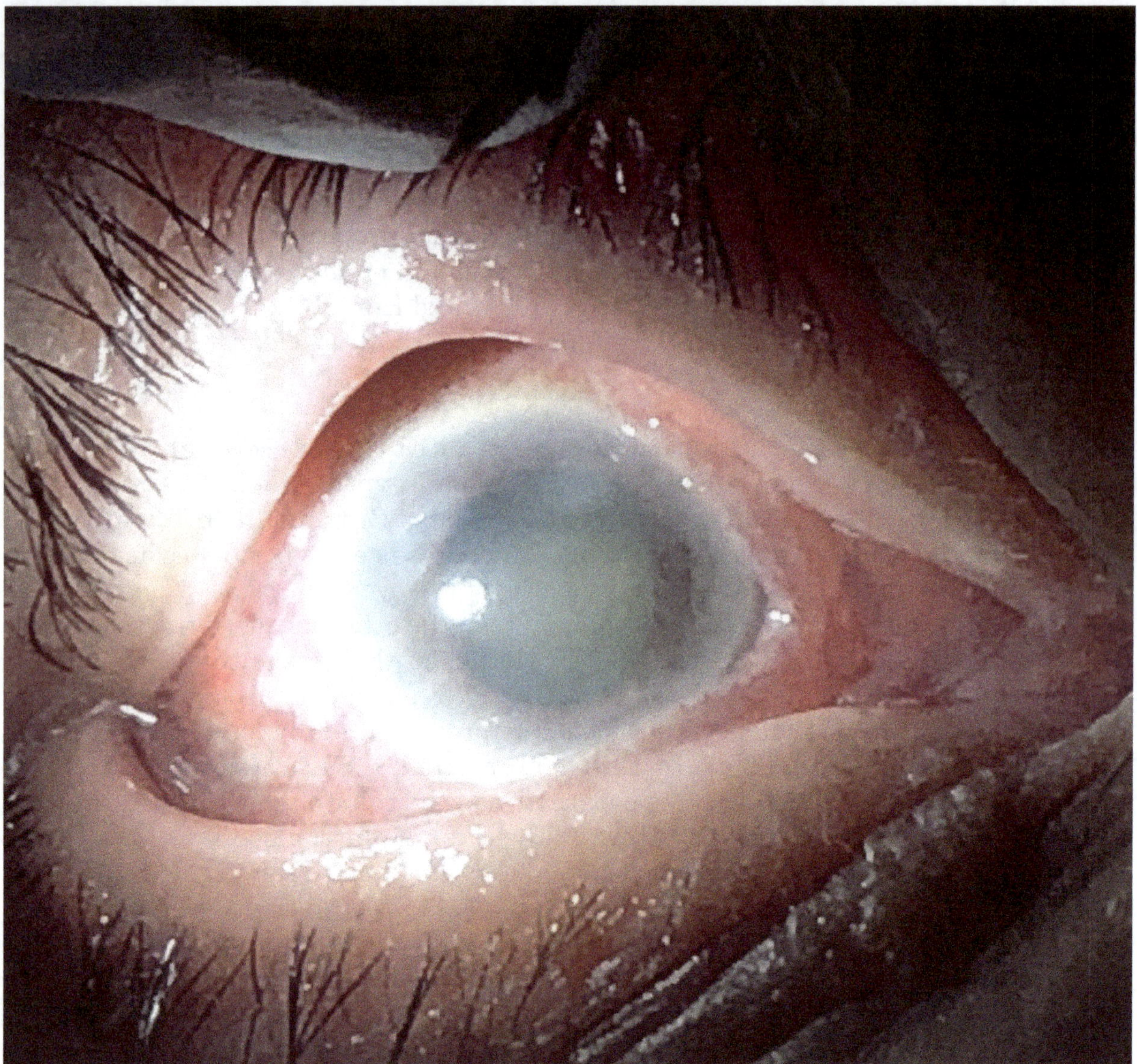

**Fig. 3.** The pupil in angle-closure glaucoma can look green when the mid-dilated pupil exposes the opalescent lens of middle age.

edema, can lighten the cornea over a large extent of its surface. In addition, the mydriasis of angle-closure glaucoma can expose the lens, which, in some cases, appears opalescent (green) or gray (Fig. 3).[110] Thus, it is not surprising that many early cultures use the term for a glaucous eye to describe such blinding conditions. In Mesoamerica, the Nahuatl treated a diseased blue or green pupil by rubbing the eye.[111] In China, blindness with a green pupil (*qing mang*) preceded the introduction of couching into the region.[112]

---

110 Leffler, Schwartz, Giliberti, et al. 2015; Leffler, Schwartz 2020b, pp. 145-196; Leffler et al. 2017.

111 Leffler et al. 2017.

112 Deshpande 1999.

Some Old World societies which came into contact with people with light blue eyes used the same term to describe a healthy light blue or green eye and the lightest category of diseased eye. In Hippocratic Greece, which was a precouching society (as far as we know), the lightest eye category was described as *glaukos,* regardless of whether the eye was a normal blue eye or a diseased eye. Although the *glaukos* eye was not consistent with good vision, the *glaukos* eye might be transient or improve, just as a keratitis might improve. It would not hurt to try medicines, though it is doubtful that ancient medicines were typically efficacious for most conditions.[113] As noted earlier, an Egyptian papyrus from the 2nd century BCE described an ophthalmic condition with a pupil described as *glaukos.*

A transition in the significance of the glaucous hue occurred as cataract couching entered a region. Eyes with extensive light areas from corneal scarring, keratitis, and so on, or those with mydriasis exposing a gray or opalescent cataract, were less likely to benefit from cataract couching; therefore, the *glaukos* hue was regarded as surgically incurable.[114]

During the medieval period, the Greek term *glaukos* was translated into Arabic as *zarqaa.* This term was analogous, because it described both the healthy light-colored blue or green eye and the diseased eye with a bright gray or green pupil.[115]

In India as well, it is possible that the same word for the healthy blue eye (*nīla*) was also used for a surgically incurable category of eye disease, as discussed in the chapter on India.

The ophthalmic chapter of Celsus mentioned two color terms which described healthy light blue eyes: *caesius* and *caeruleus.* Of the two, *caeruleus* might tend to a darker blue and, like *nīla* in the works of Suśruta, described a pupillary hue which was not treatable with couching. *Caeruleus* could also describe green objects, such as plants.[116]

Georg Bartisch in 1583 described caerulean cataracts (*Coerulea*), which were the color of indigo, "somewhat glassy," and typically did not improve with surgery.[117] Presumably, this information was an amplification of Celsus, rather than being derived directly from the Indian works.

---

113  Leffler, Schwartz 2020a, pp. 1-46.

114  Leffler, Schwartz 2020a, pp. 1-46; Leffler, Schwartz, Hadi, et al. 2015.

115  Leffler, Schwartz, Hadi, et al. 2015.

116  Leffler, Schwartz, Hadi, et al. 2015.

117  Bartisch, Blanchard 1996, p. 50.

## A Sense of Humors (50 BCE)

Both Greco-Roman and Indian works specified that the humor settling in the eye not only determined the appearance of the pupil to the doctor but also tinged the vision of the patient correspondingly. The earliest datable record of this idea comes from the Roman poet Lucretius, who wrote in 50 BCE: "…whatever jaundiced people view, becomes wan-yellow…"[118] The Romans sometimes compared jaundice to the color of gold (*aurugineus* or *aurugo*).[119] Thus, the description of one type of incurable cataract as golden in color in the works of Celsus (1st century) and Vegetius (4th century) might correspond with the idea that cataracts could be caused by bile.[120]

Of course, the idea that jaundice could be associated with ophthalmic disorders is even older. Ancient Mesopotamian medicine not only described white films in the eye but also noted that a filmy membrane could occur due to jaundice (*āmurriqanu*), in which case the membrane could be removed by daubing with a medicine.[121]

In the later Greek works, the visual impact of humors in the eye is well represented with respect to yellow bile and blood. Sextus Empiricus wrote in *Outlines of Pyrrhonism*: "Thus, sufferers from jaundice declare that objects which seem to us white are yellow, while those whose eyes are bloodshot call them blood-red…Surely, then, we have much more reason to suppose that when different juices [χυμῶν, *chymon*] are intermingled in the vision of animals their impressions of the objects will become different."[122] This is interesting because Sextus Empiricus was relating the philosophy of Pyrrho, who accompanied Alexander the Great to India, including Taxila.[123]

Others have noted similarities between the philosophy of Sextus Empriricus and the Mahayana Buddhist thinker Nagarjuna.[124] Indeed, the ophthalmic portion of the Sushruta Samhita is attributed to a figure called Nagarjuna and also describes colored entoptic phenomena.

In the Greco-Roman works, this idea continued in Galen's *On Diseases and Symptoms*:

> If the fluids…are changed in colour, a false vision (*parorasis*) involving the nature of those things occurs…those who are jaundiced seem to see everything as pale yellow but those who have suffered a hyphaema (*hyposphagma*) as red.[125]


118  Lucretius, Leonard 1921, p. 147.

119  Leverett 1837, p. 95.

120  Leffler, Schwartz, Hadi, et al. 2015.

121  Attia 2018.

122  Sextus Empiricus, Bury 1933, p. 28.

123  Beckwith 2015, pp. 13-16, 57; McEvilley 2002, p. 450; Neale 2014.

124  McEvilley 2001.

125  Galen, Johnston 2006, p. 212. (Kühn 7.99)

Likewise, Ibn Isa wrote that if the cornea is red from blood, objects appear red, but if one has jaundice, the yellow color of the cornea makes objects appear yellow.[126]

Perhaps, this teaching eventually spread to China as well. In the 14th- or 15th-century Chinese treatise *Essential Subtleties on the Silver Sea*, "blood pours into the pupil" was a disorder in which poisonous blood pours into the water of the golden well, as the pupil [is also called]…Periodically pain and roughness [are felt]. A red gleam fills the eye.[127] The translator interpreted this passage to refer to erythropsia, or red-tinged vision. The disorder was felt to result from illnesses of the liver or kidney, trauma, or improper couching.

## Mediterranean Ophthalmologists Arriving from the East (25 CE)

In contrast with the stories of Cyrus' oculist and Apollonius traveling Eastward, we could not find stories of ancient Mediterranean oculists with Persian or Indian origins. Perhaps, the closest example was the following funerary inscription: D(ecimus) Colius D(ecimi) l(ibertus) Arsaces was a *"medicus ocularius"* who practiced in Rome between 25 BCE to 25 CE, and is believed to have a Greek or Persian family name.[128]

Many years later, we hear of a Romani oculist in France. In 1465, Martin de Calera, a Romani physician ("*dc Parvo Egito*"), passing through Tarascon, signed a contract to cure the eye ailment suffered by the Jewish physician Salves Avigdor (1441-1487).[129]

## Aulus Cornelius Celsus (c. 25 BCE–c. 50 CE)

The cataract surgery description by the encyclopedist Celsus is one of the earliest, and most complete, descriptions of the procedure from antiquity:

> I have already made mention elsewhere of cataract [*suffusionis*], because when of recent origin it is also often dispersed by medicaments: when it is more chronic it requires treatment by surgery, and this is one of the most delicate operations. Before I speak of this, the nature of the eyeball itself has to be briefly explained. A knowledge of this is often useful, but especially here. The eyeball, then, has two external tunics, of which the outer is called by the Greeks *ceratoides.* In that part of the eye which is white [*alba*] it is fairly thick; over the region of the pupil [*pupillae*] it is thin. To this tunic the under one is joined; in the middle where the pupil [*pupilla*]

---

126 Ibn Isa, Wood 1936, p. 165.

127 Kovacs, Unschuld 1998, pp. 199-200. *Yin-hai jing-wei.* Disorder N25.

128 Nutton 1972, p. 20, n. 27; Cacciapuoti 2017, n. 17.

129 Wickersheimer 1936, vol. 2, pp. 540, 730.

is, it is pierced by a small hole: around this it is thin, further out it too is thicker and is called by the Greeks *chorioides*. These two tunics whilst enclosing the contents of the eyeball, coalesce again behind it, and after becoming thinned out and fused into one, go through the space between the bones, and adhere to the membrane of the brain. Under these two tunics, at the spot where the pupil is, there is an empty space [*locus vacuus*]; then underneath again is the thinnest tunic, which Herophilus named *arachnoidem*. At its middle the arachnoides is cupped, and contained in that hollow is what, from its resemblance to glass [*vitri*], the Greeks call *hyaloides*; it is humour, neither fluid nor thick, but as it were curdled, and upon its colour is dependent the colour of the pupil, whether black [*niger*] or blue [*caesius*], since the outer tunic is quite white [*alba*]: but this humour is enclosed by that thin membrane which comes over it from the interior. In front of these is a drop of humour like white of egg [*ovi albo*], from which comes the faculty of seeing; it is named by the Greeks *crystalloides*.

Now either from disease or from a blow, a humour forms underneath the two tunics in what I have stated to be an empty space [*locum esse vacuum*]; and this as it gradually hardens [*indurescens*] is an obstacle to the visual power within. And there are several species of this lesion; some curable, some which do not admit of treatment. For there is hope if the cataract [*suffusio*] is small, and immobile, if it has also the colour of sea water [*marinae aquae*] or of glistening iron [*ferri nitentis*], and if at the side there persists some sensation to a flash of light. If large, if the black [*nigra*] part of the eye has lost its natural configuration and is changed to another form, if the colour of the suffusion is blue [*caeruleus*] or golden [*auri*], if it shakes and moves this way and that, then it is scarcely ever to be remedied. Generally too the case is worse when the cataract has arisen from a severe disease, from severe pains in the head or from a blow of a violent kind. Old age is not favourable for treatment, since apart from this lesion, sharpness of vision is naturally dulled; neither is childhood favourable, but rather intermediate ages. Neither a small nor a sunken eye is satisfactory for treatment. And in the cataract itself, there is a certain development [*maturitas*]. Therefore we must wait until it is no longer fluid, but appears to have coalesced to some sort of hardness [*duritie*]. Before treatment the patient should eat in moderation and for three days beforehand drink water, for the day before abstain from everything. After these preparations, he is to be seated in a light place [*loco lucido*], with his face towards the light [*lumine*], in such a manner that the physician may sit opposite to him, a little more elevated; the assistant from behind holds the head so that the patient does not move: for vision can be destroyed permanently by a slight movement. In order also that the eye to be treated may be held more still, wool [*lana*] is put over the opposite eye and bandaged on: further the left eye should be operated on with the right hand, and the right eye with the left hand. Thereupon a needle [*acus*] is to be taken pointed enough to penetrate, yet not too fine; and this is to be inserted straight through the two outer tunics at a point intermediate between the pupil of the eye and the angle adjacent to the temple, [*medio loco inter oculi nigrum et angulum tempori propiorem*] away from the middle of the cataract, in such a way that no vein [*vena*] is wounded. The needle should not be, however, entered timidly, for it passes into the empty space; [*inani loco excipitur*] and when this is reached even a man of moderate experience cannot be mistaken, for there is then no resistance to pressure. When the spot is reached, the needle is to be sloped against the suffusion itself and should gently rotate there and little by little guide it below the region of the pupil; when the cataract has passed below the pupil it is pressed upon most firmly in order that it may settle below. If it sticks there the cure is accomplished; if it returns to some extent, it is to be cut up with the same needle and separated into several pieces, which can be the more easily stowed away singly, and form smaller obstacles to vision. After this the needle is drawn straight out; and soft wool [*lana*] soaked in white of egg [*ovi album*] is to be put on, and above this something to check inflammation; and then bandages. Subsequently the patient must have rest, abstinence, and inunction with soothing medicaments; the day following will be soon enough for food, which at first should be liquid to avoid the use of the jaws; then, when the inflammation is over, such as has been prescribed for wounds, and in addition to these directions it is necessary that water should for some time be the only drink.[130]

It is not clear that Celsus actually performed the procedure.

## Intermediate Age of the Patient (50 CE)

Both Greco-Roman and Ayurvedic works recommended cataract surgery on patients of intermediate ages. In the work of Celsus, intermediate ages were preferred, and the older patients were thought to have worse outcomes because "apart from this lesion [suffusions], sharpness of vision is naturally dulled." The Biblical story of healing a man born blind seems to indicate some awareness among laypeople along the Mediterranean of the difficulty of treating congenital vision loss (John 9:32).[131] Earlier, Celsus had noted with respect to letting blood that "the ancients were of opinion that the first and last years could not sustain this kind of treatment."[132] As in the Indian works, the concern was weakness of the patient. In contrast with those he called the "ancients," Celsus based the decision for bloodletting on an evaluation of the strength of the individual patient. Hippocrates in the latter (older) portion of *Diseases 2* had already advised in the treatment of various medical conditions: "draw blood from his arms, unless he is weak."[133] Galen advised: "If [the patient] is either a child or an old person, phlebotomy is ruled out. But between these ages, when bodily strength is present in the patient, you must carry out phlebotomy…"[134]

---

130 Celsus, Spencer 1938, vol. III, pp. 345-353. (7.7.13-14). Translations of *ferri nitentis* (polished iron) and sentence on patient in a "light place" are from Celsus, Lee 1831, vol. I, pp. 259-260. *Caesius* and *caeruleus* were translated simply as blue, as informed by our prior analyses of ancient color terms.

131 Leffler, Schwartz, Davenport, 2014.

132 Celsus, Spencer 1935, vol. 1, p. 155. (2.10.1)

133 Hippocrates, Potter 1988, p. 291. (Littré VII 112)

134 Galen et al. 2011, pp. 398-399. Method of Medicine VIII. Kühn 10.565.

The Ayurvedic works also indirectly recommended cataract couching on patients of intermediate ages, but not in a way that indicated an awareness of the potential for amblyopia in the young or coexisting visual disorders in the older patients. The cataract surgery chapter in the *Suśrutasamhita* noted: "Persons declared unfit for venesection (viz., infants, old men, etc.) in the chapter on venesection should not be subjected to any surgical operation."[135] This prohibition in children was not because of a concern for amblyopia. Rather, the concern expressed in the earlier volume was that the young and old would be too weak to tolerate a procedure.[136] The earlier volume noted that because leech application was the most delicate method of letting blood, it was suitable for "children, old, timid, debilitated" patients.[137] Likewise, cauterization was also prohibited in "debilitated, child, old, timid" patients.[138] In contrast with the Ayurvedic works, the Buddhist sutras did evince an understanding of amblyopia.


## Maturity of the Cataract (30 CE)

The crystalline lens hardens as a person ages, and when it is couched while very soft, it breaks up, rather than moving into the vitreous intact. Evaluating the hardness, or maturity, of the cataract was found in the earliest Indo-Greek writings of Celsus and Suśruta.[139] Eventually, it came to incorporate more primitive doctrines of evaluation of pupillary color, rubbing the eye, and blowing on the eye.


## Patient Positioning and Environment (30 CE)

The common denominator for almost all couching stories, whether from the east or the west, is that the patient is sitting upright (Figs. 4A, 4B).[140] This upright position is present in the early accounts of Celsus and the Sushruta Samhita and continues through the medieval, and into the modern period. In the early European writings, such as the work of Celsus, the patient is described as sitting lower than the doctor.

The near universal use of having the patient sitting upright probably stems from the fact that gravity can assist with displacing the lens into the inferior part of the

---

135 Sushruta, Bhishagratna 1916, vol. 3, p. 79.

136 Susruta, Sharma 2018, vol. 1, p. 134.

137 Susruta, Sharma 2018, vol. 1, p. 134.

138 Susruta, Sharma 2018, vol. 1, p. 127.

139 Celsus wrote: "And in the cataract itself, there is a certain development. Therefore we must wait until it is no longer fluid, but appears to have coalesced to some sort of hardness."(-Celsus, Spencer 1938, vol. 3, p. 347) (7.7.14) *Suśrutasaṃhitā* 6.17.79 noted that "The disorder occurs [...] also if punctured in too immature [*taruṇa-*] stage" (Suśruta, Sharma 2014, vol. 3, p. 206; No author listed. Digital Corpus of Sanskrit 2020) Likewise, the *Aṣṭāṅgahṛdayasaṃhitā* noted that couching for cataract (liṅganāśa) is performed when it is due to kapha and is ripe (sujāta) (Meulenbeld 1999, vol. 1A, p. 450).

140 Rambo 1955. Mishima 2004, p. 64.

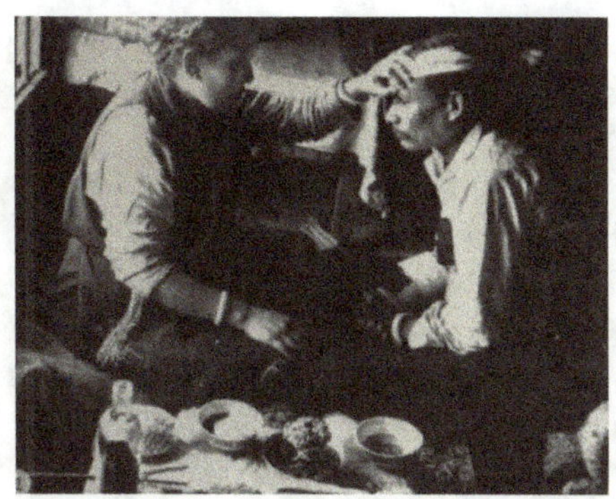

**Fig. 4A.** A woman oculist from Tibet examines a man's eye before she couches his cataract, in 1955. Both doctor and patient sit on the floor. The patient's contralateral eye is covered.

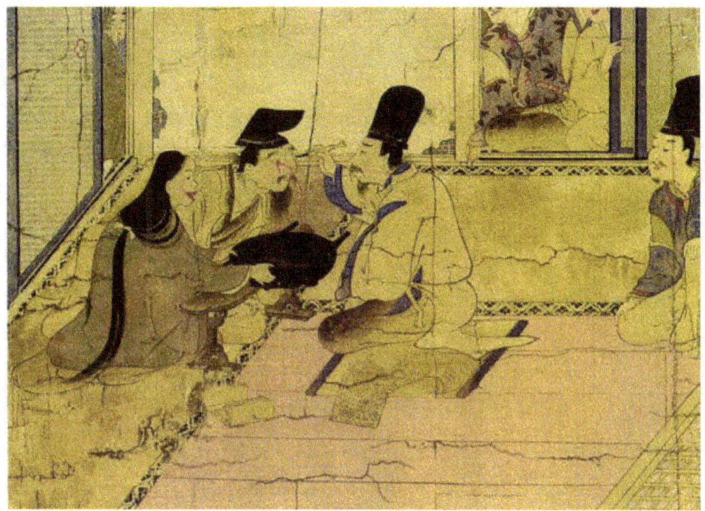

**Fig. 4B.** Picture of an unsuccessful needling procedure of the eye of a man from Nara, in Yamai no Sôshi, Japan, by Tosa Mitsunaga, dated to the end of the Heian Era, about 1184 CE (Mishima 2004, p. 64).

eye, out of the visual axis. If the patient were supine, the lens could fall onto the macula, but would still remain in the visual axis. The rare medieval account of a cataract couching performed supine is the exception, which merely proves the rule (Fig. 4C).[141] In contrast, Celsus would allow the pterygium patient to be supine or sitting, depending on which eye was being treated.[142]

The early writings from the early Mediterranean are somewhat ambiguous about whether the surgery is performed inside or outside. Celsus did not mention the breeze and referred merely to light, rather than sun. Celsus' word for place, *loco*, could be either a room or an outdoor location. The ophthalmic healing stories of Jesus in a

---

141 Mishima 2004, p. 78.
142 Celsus, Spencer 1938, vol. 3, p. 328.

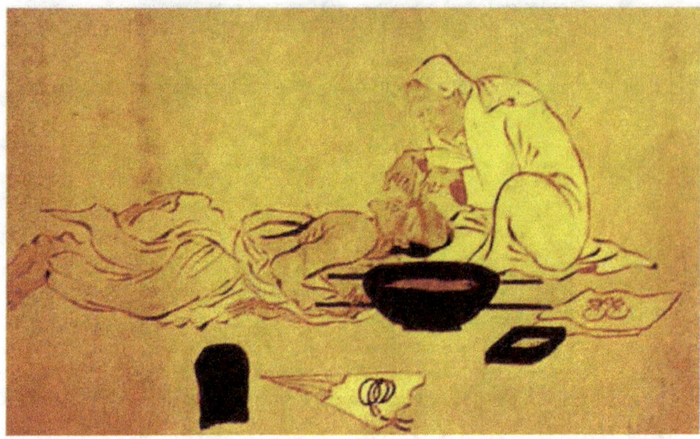

**Fig. 4C.** An ophthalmic procedure said to be cataract couching, with the patient supine, from Japan in the 13th century (Mishima 2004, p. 78).

temple or a home, the Temple of Asclepius, Vespasian at the Temple of Serapis, Ananias treating St. Paul in a home, Apollonius in temples, and a fresco of Saint Colluthos all suggest that ophthalmic healing could have been performed indoors.

On the other hand, we also have evidence of ophthalmic healing along the Mediterranean performed outside, such as the Tomb of Ipwy, the story of Tobit, and some of Jesus' healings.

In all writings, from Celsus onward, the patient is looking in the direction of the light (or the sun). This probably stems from the need for the operator to have adequate lighting to accomplish the task. In addition, in the early works of Celsus and Suśruta, an assistant holds the patient's head during cataract surgery.[143]

Ancient writings do not describe cataract patients standing. Indeed, a standing posture would seem to be very unstable. Still, some images seem to depict ophthalmic healing performed with the doctor or the patient standing. Ancient Roman funerary images have a doctor standing in front of a sitting patient, or both the doctor and the patient standing (Figs. 5, 6).[144]

---

143  Breton 1826.
144  Gasson 1986, Baker 2011.

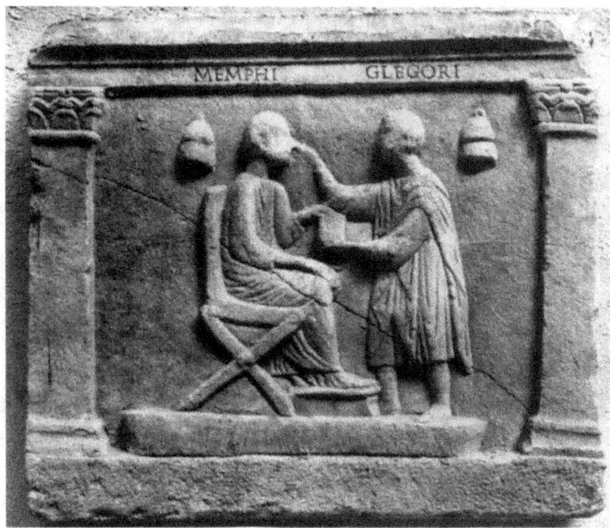

**Fig. 5.** An oculist standing while treating a seated patient, depicted on a sarcophagus of the Sosia family (3rd-4th centuries CE) at the church of San Vittore, Ravenna.

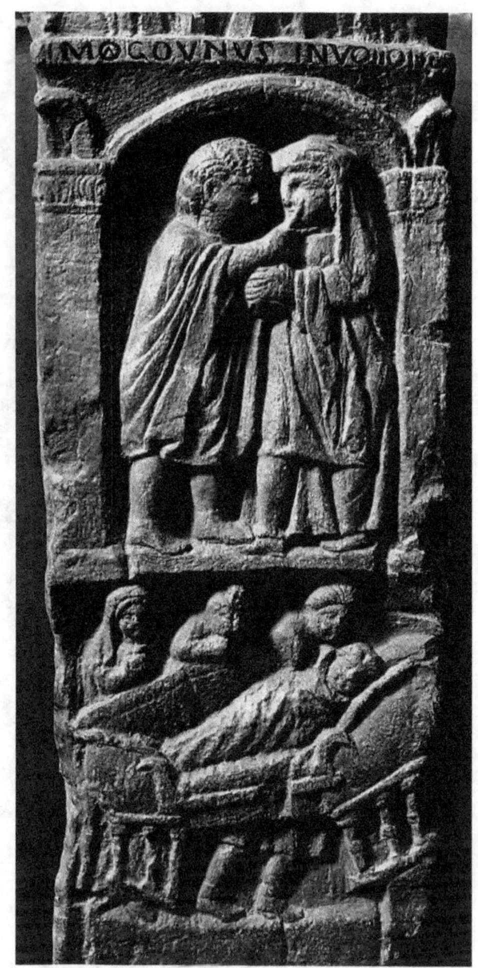

**Fig. 6.** Funerary relief from Gallia Belgica possibly depicting eye surgery or the application of a medicine, with both the doctor and the patient standing (Belgica CIL XIII 4668).

A fresco from about 800 CE in the Deir al-Surian monastery in the Scetis Desert in Egypt shows Saint Colluthos sitting while performing an eye surgery on a standing patient and is realistic and detailed enough to suggest that the artist was familiar with cataract couching, although other types of ophthalmic healing cannot be excluded (Fig. 7).[145]

Finally, images from England and the low countries in the 12th century depict both the doctor and the patient standing. A manuscript showing a couching in Tournai in 1351 shows the oculist standing in front of the sitting patient. All of the images with the patient standing are highly stylized and may be abstract representations

---

145 Starodubcev 2018.

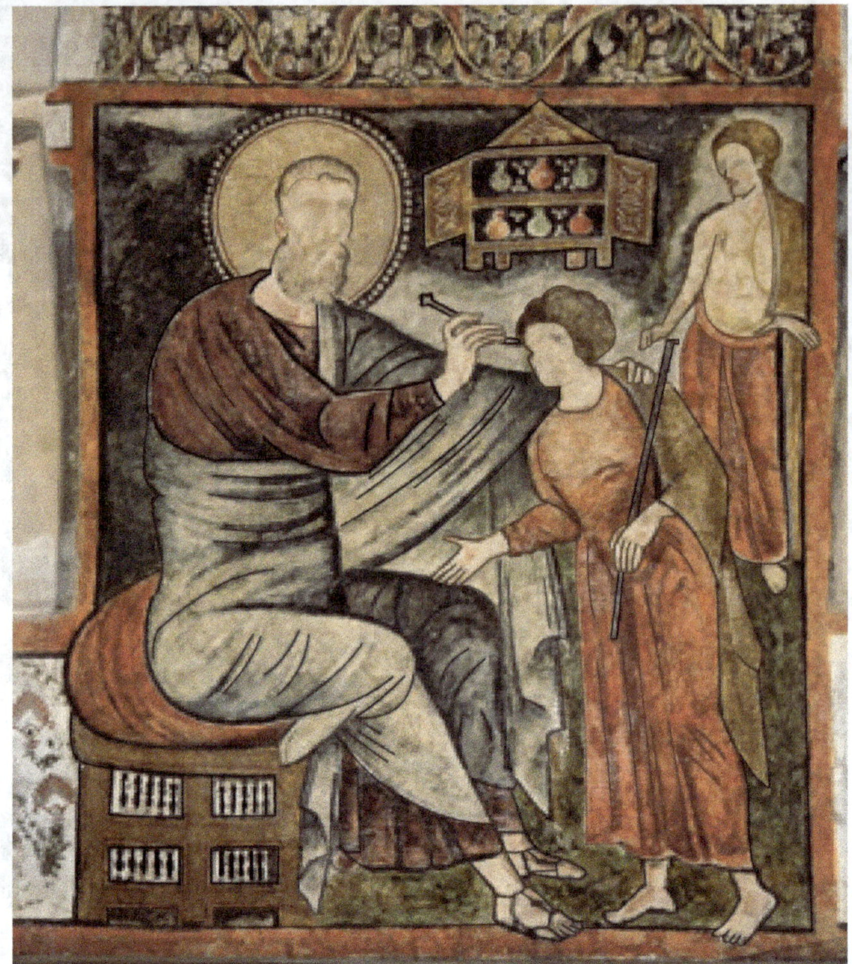

**Fig. 7.** A frescoe from 800 CE in the Deir al-Surian monastery in the Scetis Desert in Egypt shows Saint Colluthos sitting while performing an eye surgery.

by nonmedical illustrators. Moreover, even if they do represent ophthalmic healing, which is not always clear, they could represent procedures other than cataract surgery.

We did find that in 1824, an Irish ophthalmologist named Edward Fitzgerald encountered a 60-year-old man in San Pablo, Mexico, and performed a cataract extraction in the street with both the doctor and the patient standing, and the patient's back up against a wall.[146] Therefore, having a patient stand during cataract surgery is not impossible.

The works of Antyllus (approximately 3rd century) introduce two new aspects regarding the lighting. First, the light source toward which the patient is turned is specified as the sun, which indicates that the patient is probably outside. Second,

---

146 Leffler, Wainsztein 2016.

Antyllus and subsequent authors advise that the patient is in a shadow, rather than directly in the sun.[147] Presumably, one wanted to avoid so much light that the pupil was constricted. In fact, in some of al-Rāzī's accounts, the statement that the cataract is seen better if direct sunlight is avoided seems to be attributed to Antyllus. The explicit statement that light constricts the pupil is found in the Ayurvedic works of Vāgbhata, and in some (but not all) of the manuscripts of the Sushruta Samhita.[148] Paulus Aegineta in the 6th century provided similar instructions.[149]

The Sushruta Samhita of the early Common Era, and related Ayurvedic works, had recommended performing cataract couching at a season that was neither too hot nor too cold. However, a different approach is observed beginning with *Sapientia Artis Medicinae* of 6th-century Europe. In short, the medieval works advised against a cold breeze blowing into the patient's face. Mentioning the breeze is important, in part, because it is additional evidence that the procedure was performed outside. In *Sapientia Artis Medicinae*, one performed couching in May, the summer, or the fall. In other words, one did not need to avoid the hottest weather.

Cataract surgery during the summer is also recommended in Ibn Isa's text of 11th-century Baghdad:

> ...let him be seated in shadow but facing the light. Choose a northern exposure [a day with wind from the North], and preferably, a summer's day...The patient should sit on a soft pillow; bind his knees together in front of his body, also tie his hands to one another and to his thighs. You should sit on a chair (or stool) correspondingly higher (than the patient)...During the operation an assistant should stand behind the patient and hold his head.[150]

Ibn Isa literally writes that one chooses a "northern day," and this wording has flummoxed translators. Elsewhere in this volume, Mathias Witt solves this puzzle by noting that Ṣalāḥ al-Dīn al-Kaḥḥāl of 13th-century Hama, Syria stated that the cataract should be operated on a day with Northern air (*i.e.* wind) rather than southern air, and so Witt postulates that the available manuscript of Ibn Isa's treatise is missing the word "air." In the Northern hemisphere, a patient facing the sun will be facing south. Indeed, the southward-facing posture is confirmed in the Chinese literature (see later). If the wind is coming from the North, it will not be blowing directly in the patient's face.

---

147 "Antilis: For the cataract operation the patient is seated in a shadow and faces the sun. The head of the patient is held firmly..."(Hirschberg, Blodi 1982, vol. 1, p. 348)

148 See chapter on pupillary responses, and Mathias Witt's chapter on Antyllus.

149 Paulus, Adams 1846, vol. 2, p. 280. "...having placed the patient opposite the light, but not in the sun..."

150 Ibn Isa, Wood 1936, pp. 184-185. Hirschberg provides an alternative understanding, by indicating that in a Dresden manuscript of Ibn Isa, the text reads: "The day should be one of the northern sun and not of the southern sun" (Hirschberg, Blodi 1985, vol. 2, p. 218). In the Northern hemisphere, the sun is located more Northerly in the sky around the summer solstice (about June 21). Therefore, this text would suggest surgery in the Spring or Summer.

In the Ayurvedic literature, the breeze on the operative day is not mentioned until the *Aṣṭāṅgasaṃgraha* (AS) of Vāgbhata I in the 7th century, which indicated that cataract surgery should be performed:

> On an auspicious day, both the patient and the physician having performed auspicious rites, offered prayers to Āditya (the sun) and Videhādhipati (king of Videha) in the morning, select a place devoid of breeze and bright light, make the patient sit on a soft bed spread on the ground facing the sun, extending both his legs, placing the palms of both his hands firmly on the ground.[151]

In China, the teaching was also found in the early 9th-century *Treatise of Bodhisattva Nagarjuna on Eye (Diseases)*:

> On the day of the operation, the weather should be clear with soft wind and a bright day that removes darkness and confusion...also the weather should be warm...Let the patient face south and catch the doctor by the waist.[152]

Likewise, the 14th-century Chinese treatise *Essential Subtleties on the Silver Sea* recommended:

> For all golden-needle surgery one must choose an auspicious day. The wind should be still, and it should be a warm day.[153]

Abū al-Qāsim Khalaf ibn al-'Abbās al-Zahrāwī al-Ansari (936-1013 CE), known later as Albucasis, did not know about avoiding direct sunlight: "You should advise the patient to sit down cross-legged before you, facing the light in full sun..."[154]

Khalifah of 13th-century Aleppo advised:

> The patient should then be seated in the shade, facing the light. He should sit facing the sun...Let the patient sit on a cushion. Bring his knees in close to his chest and have him hold his thighs together with both hands. You sit on a chair somewhat higher than the patient.[155]

---

151 Vāgbhata, Murthy 2000, p. 150.

152 Deshpande, Fan "Restoring the Dragon's Vision" 2012, p 110. Treatise: *Longshu pusa yanlun*.

153 Kovacs, Unschuld 1998, p. 404. Treatise: *Yin-hai jing-wei*.

154 Albucasis et al. 1973, p. 252.

155 Blodi et al. 1993, p. 215.

# Using Both Hands: Ambidexterity (30 CE)

From the ancient Mediterranean and India to medieval China, the healer was required to be ambidextrous. The right hand was used to couch the cataract in the left eye, and the left hand was used to couch the cataract in the right eye. Perhaps, there is no "smoking gun" to establish that cataract surgery originated close to the Mediterranean. However, if there is a smoking gun, it might be this emphasis on ambidexterity, which had always been favored by the Greeks. Homer wrote in the *Iliad* that "the warrior Asteropaeus hurled with both spears at once, since he was ambidextrous [περιδέξιος, *peridexios*]."[156] In the 6th century BCE, the poet Hipponax wrote: "for I have two right hands [ἀμφιδέξιος, *amphidexios*] and I don't miss with my Punches."[157] Hippocrates in *Aphorisms* insisted: "A woman does not become ambidextrous [ἀμφιδέξιος, *amphidexios*]."[158] Also, the Hippocratic work *In the Surgery* emphasized: "The hands of the operator must be so skilled that he is able to execute without further operative manipulation, that is be ambidextrous."[159] Plato in *Laws VII* praised the Scythian warriors, who with bow and arrow could "use either hand for both purposes."[160] The Old Testament figure Ehud had a right hand that was "bound," which might have indicated that he had been trained to use his left hand. Ehud was able to stab the Moabite king using his left hand (Judges 3:12-26). The Septuagint, the Greek translation of the Bible from Egypt in the 3rd and 2nd centuries BCE, described Ehud as ἀμφοτεροδέξιος (*amphoterodexios*), which has been translated as "ambidextrous."[161] Aristotle wrote in *Historia Animalium II*: "Man is the only animal which can actually become ambidextrous [ἀμφιδέξιον, *amphidexion*]."[162] He also wrote in *Nicomachean Ethics*: "By nature the right hand is stronger, yet it is possible that all men should come to be ambidextrous."[163] Finally, in the 6th century CE, Procopius of Caesarea related that the warrior Althias caught a spear with his right hand, "And with his left hand he drew his bow instantly, for he was ambidextrous [ἀμφιδέξιος, *amphidexios*]."[164]

---

156 Homer, Murray 1925, p. 416.

157 Iliad 21. Archilochus, Semonides, Hipponax, Gerber DE (trans.) 1999, p. 452.

158 Hippocrates, Jones 1931, p. 202.

159 In the surgery, Κατ ιητρειον (*Kat Ietreion*). Magnus, Waugh 1998, part. 1, p. 127.

160 Plato, Jowett 1871, vol. 4, p. 308.

161 Ausloos 2017.

162 Aristotle, Peck 1965, p. 76.

163 Remow, Aristotle 2008, pp. 585-600.

164 Procopius, Dewing 1916, pp. 318.

Ambidexterity was required in cataract surgery because a temporal approach was favored. In the cataract description of Celsus, "the left eye should be operated on with the right hand, and the right eye with the left hand."[165] Likewise, Paulus Aegineta, recording Galen's method, wrote: "…if it is the left eye we operate with the right hand, or if the left eye with the right…"[166] Albucasis also advised ambidexterity, operating with the ipsilateral hand.[167]

In Celsus' work, ambidexterity was praised beyond the cataract operation. In general, Celsus noted that the good surgeon was "ready to use the left hand as well as the right."[168] Celsus recommended when sewing abdominal wounds that "…the surgeon's left hand pushes the needle from within outwards through the right margin of the wound, and his right hand through the left margin…"[169] On the other hand, for pterygium surgery, Celsus was willing to move the patient to prevent the surgeon having to switch hands.[170]

Many of the religious ophthalmic cures are specified as requiring the use of both of the healer's hands. Tobit's son performed the healing in such a manner: "And he scaled it off with both hands from the corner of his eyes." The Gospel of Acts described that Saint Paul "has seen in a vision a man named Ananias come in and lay his hands on him, so that he might regain his sight." Later, Ananias did effect the cure by "laying his hands on him." Likewise, the Gospel of Mark specified that when curing the blind man at Bethsaida, Jesus "laid his hands upon him."[171]

The advocacy of ambidexterity appears to have spread Eastward and is found in the Ayurvedic works, as early as the Sushruta Samhita.[172] This practice might have been copied from the Greeks. Outside cataract surgery, Indian literature generally gave special significance to the use of each hand, with the right hand suited for some tasks and the left hand suited for others.

Of note, one early Chinese work (*Longshu pusa yanlun, Treatise of Bodhisattva Nagarjuna on Eye (Diseases)*) of the early 9th century recommended a temporal approach and surgical ambidexterity.[173] However, no mention of the hand used survived in a 14th- or 15th-century Chinese text.[174]

---

165 Celsus 7.7.14. Celsus, Spencer 1938, vol. 3, p. 350.

166 Paulus Aegineta, Adams 1846, vol. 2, p. 280.

167 Albucasis et al. 1973, p. 252.

168 Celsus 7.0.4. Celsus, Spencer 1938, vol. 3, p. 296.

169 Celsus 7.16.4. Celsus, Spencer 1938, vol. 3, p. 386.

170 Celsus, Spencer 1938, vol. 3, p. 328.

171 This contrasts with the corresponding otolaryngologic healing in Mark (7:32-6) in which just one hand was used, and we read: "…one that was deaf, and had an impediment in his speech; and they beseech him to lay his hand upon him."

172 Leffler, Klebanov et al. 2020.

173 Deshpande, Fan "Restoring the Dragon's Vision" 2012, p. 111.

174 Kovacs, Unschuld 1998, pp. 404-405. Essential Subtleties on the Silver Sea, *Yin-hai jing-wei*.

# Pars Plana Puncture Avoiding Vessels (30 CE)

In the Indo-Greek works, couching is performed with pars plana entry of a needle or rod, making sure to avoid blood vessels (Figs. 8A, 8B).[175] In the earliest Roman work (Celsus) and earliest Indian works (Suśruta and Vāgbhaṭa), the primary instrument (needle or rod) is directly applied to, and punctures, the sclera at the pars plana. A detailed analysis of the early Greco-Roman works (Celsus, pseudo-Galen, and Paulus Aegineta), supported by experiments, confirmed that the approach was pars plana.[176] For Celsus, the needle penetrated at an intermediate point between the limbus and the external canthus, which many people have interpreted to be at the half-way point, though the original text is not completely specific.[177]

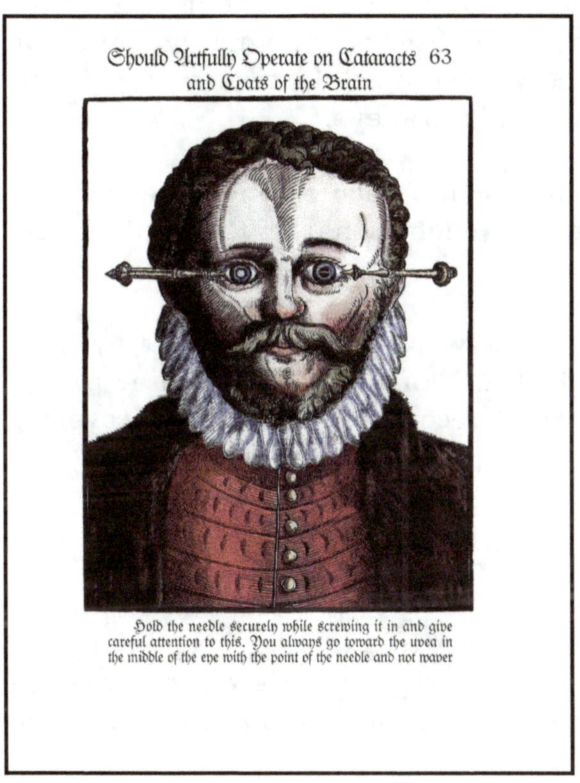


**Fig. 8A.** The couching needle enters the pars plana and passes posterior to the iris from the 1583 ophthalmic treatise of Georg Bartisch.

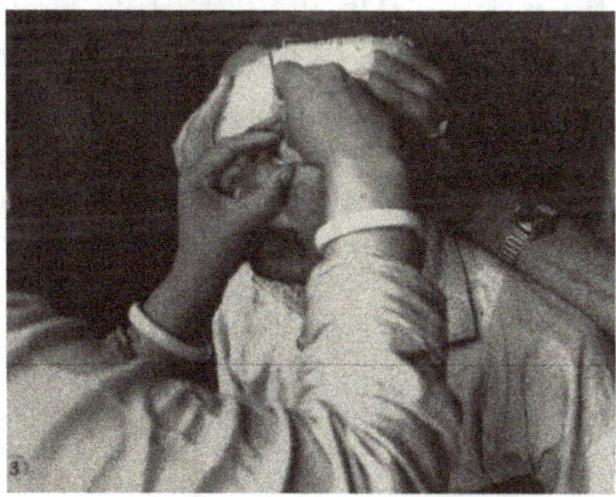

**Fig. 8B.** The couching needle approaches from the temporal side, seen in Tibet in 1955. The contralateral eye is covered.

---

175 Breton 1826.

176 Leffler, Hadi, et al. 2016.

177 Celsus (7.7.14). Celsus, Spencer 1938, vol. 3, p. 350.

The distance from the limbus to the lateral canthus was on average 9.0 mm in adults when we conducted experiments and asked them to gaze straight ahead (because no other direction of gaze is specified in the above Greco-Roman works). If the puncture were at half the distance, it would be at 4.5 mm, whereas the pars plana extends to about 6 mm posterior to the limbus.[178] Avoidance of the blood vessels during surgery is found in both Celsus and the Ayurvedic works.[179]

## Covering the Nonoperative Eye (30 CE)

As early as the works of Celsus and Paulus, the Greco-Roman works recommended covering the nonoperative eye.[180] Albucasis of the 10th century and Benevenutus Grassus of the 12th or 13th century continued this Mediterranean tradition of patching (or closing) the nonoperative eye without asking the patient to converge the eyes.[181] Ibn Isa combined the Mediterranean tradition of patching the sound eye with the tradition of asking the patient to gaze at the nose.[182] Benevenutus Grassus in the 12th or 13th century also closed the contralateral eye.

Perhaps, closing the sound eye as a therapeutic approach extended beyond cataract surgery. Demosthenes Philalethes wrote: "When a gnat or other insect gets into the eye, the sound eye should be closed..."[183]

This practice of contralateral patching spread eastward into India so that, by 1824, Breton was able to observe the practice in Calcutta.[184] Like Ibn Isa, this practitioner also had the patient gaze toward the nose. The Greco-Roman practice of covering the nonoperative eye had arrived in Tibet by the 20th century (Fig. 9).[185]

## Entering an Empty Space (30 CE)

One important concept in Greco-Roman ophthalmology that has figured prominently in the 20th-century scholarship is that when the needle has entered the eye completely, one comes to an empty space. Celsus stated explicitly that he mentioned

---

178　Leffler, Hadi, et al. 2016.

179　Celsus advised that when making counter openings for missile removal, "no vein...nor an artery is cut" (7.5.1); when perforating dropsical patients "no blood vessel is cut into" (7.15.1); when advancing foreskin over the glans "great care is taken not to cut into...the blood vessels" (7.25.1); and finally, when incising an abscess under the tongue "no large blood vessel is cut into" (7.12.5) (102).

180　Celsus (7.7.14) (Celsus, Spencer 1938, vol. 3, p. 350; Paulus, Adams 1846, vol. 2, p. 280).

181　Albucasis et al. 1973, p. 252; Leffler, Schwartz, Davenport, et al. 2014.

182　Ibn Isa, Wood 1936, p. 184.

183　Shastid 1917, vol. 11, pp. 8642-8643.

184　Breton 1826.

185　Rambo 1955.

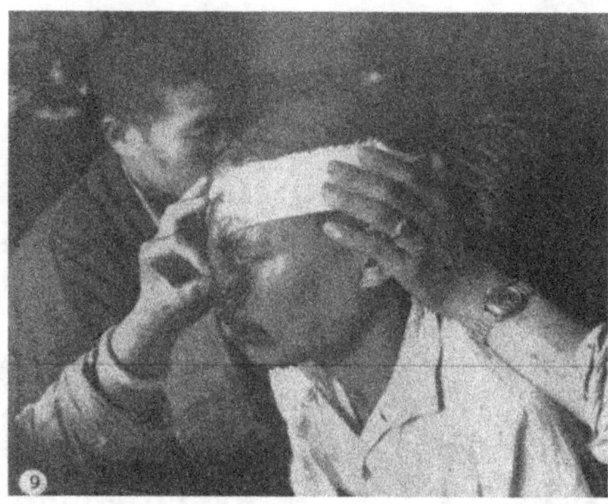

**Fig. 9.** The contralateral eye is still covered at the end of the couching procedure in Tibet in 1955. The oculist had used the right hand to displace the lens and the left hand to withdraw the needle.

this fact to indicate that there was decreased scleral resistance once the needle had penetrated the sclera. Paulus and pseudo-Galen also advised entry of the needle until it reached an empty space.[186]

The Arabic authors also mentioned this empty space. For instance, Ibn Isa wrote that one would "...push the needle towards the opposite and corresponding part of the eye until you feel that you have reached a roomy space within the eye."[187] Ammar of Cairo wrote: "When you now feel that the needle has now entered a wide space..."[188] Ibn Sina wrote that when passing the instrument, "you will reach an empty place that is vestibule-like."[189] Thus, the mention of the empty space was simply to alert the operator to expect decreased scleral resistance to the needle (as noted by Celsus) and to see the instrument in the pupil (as noted by Paulus Aegineta).

In 1901, the historian Hugo Magnus proposed that Celsus' mention of the empty space might suggest that, in contrast with Galen and Rufus, Celsus believed the lens to be in the center of the eye and could have inspired the medieval Arabic authors to accept this fallacy. In fact, there is no evidence that the medieval Arabic authors read Celsus. Moreover, Celsus' writings are consistent with the other Greek authors who mentioned the empty space entered during couching but still understood that the lens is anterior enough to touch the iris and that the peripheral lens attaches close to the corneal limbus.[190] The fallacy of the central lens seems to have originated in medieval Baghdad, in the 9th-century writings of Hunain.[191]

---

186 Leffler, Hadi, et al. 2016.

187 Ibn Isa, Wood 1936, p. 184.

188 Blodi et al. 1993, p. 153.

189 Ibn Sina, Sardo 2014, vol. 3, p. 273.

190 Shastid 1913, vol. XI, p. 8580.

191 Leffler, Hadi, et al. 2016, p. 188.

# Discission (30 CE)

Intentional discission (division) of the cataract is found in the Greco-Roman works. Celsus wrote that the operator attempted discission if the cataract failed to remain depressed. Galen wrote in *Method of Medicine XIV*:

> Apart from those, there are also some of them (I speak of the *hypochymas* [ὑποχυμάτων, *hypochymaton*]) that are more wheylike than watery. Also, those that have been pierced on all sides are dissolved straightaway, although a short time later it is as if some slime passes off below.[192]

We agree with those who believe this could represent discission (*e.g.* Lascaratos), though Hirschberg disputed this interpretation and suggested that the piercing was just of the eye, rather than the lens capsule.[193]

Ammar of Cairo recounted the case of a 30-year-old man with bilateral cataracts, the couching of one of which turned into a discission: "So I attacked the cataract with the needle vigorously. Behold, it had been cut to pieces like the membrane in an egg that encloses the white inside it."[194] Ammar wrote that the man could see afterward.

Khalifah of 13th-century Aleppo advised:

> The cataract may create problems by rising again and again as soon as the pressure is slackened off. Then break the cataract up and disperse it in all directions, upwards and downwards, and towards both canthi.[195]

Discission is mentioned in the Ayurvedic and Chinese works, but whether this was performed intentionally, or just happened to occur in soft cataracts, is less clear. The *Aṣṭāṅgasaṃgraha* recommended: "That *liṅganāśa* which breaks/splits when touched by the *śalākā* (instrument) should be given fomentation by steamcooked leaves of eranda and cleaned…"[196]

In the Chinese *Treatise of Bodhisattva Nagarjuna on Eye (Diseases)*, discission is said to occur for superficial cataracts:

> If the obstruction is superficial, then needle below it and at a distance. If the screen is turned then it exceedingly breaks down (or turn it and break it into fine pieces?).[197]

---

192 Galen et al. 2011, LCL 518, p. 534. Kühn 10.1019-20.

193 Hirschberg, Blodi 1982, vol. 1, p. 289.

194 Blodi et al. 1993, p. 161.

195 Blodi et al. 1993, p. 220.

196 Vāgbhata, Murthy 2000, vol. 3, p. 155. (*Aṣṭāṅgasaṃgraha* 6.17.25)

197 Deshpande, Fan 2012, "Restoring the Dragon's Vision," p. 110. *Longshu pusa yanlun.*

# The Blindness of Saint Paul (34 CE)

Saint Paul was cured of blindness several years after the death and resurrection of Jesus of Nazareth. This cure is distinctive because it is the only record of ophthalmic healing during the ancient Greco-Roman period in a historical person. Therefore, there is some long-term follow-up of the patient, and the story was preserved not to glorify the healer but also because of the impact the healing had on the patient.

Paul's story was told in the Acts of the Apostles. Paul was originally named Saul. He was traveling from Jerusalem to Damascus in 34 CE when he and his fellow travelers saw a light coming from heaven and heard a noise, and he was suddenly struck blind.[198] There are various alternate medical theories which could account for his symptoms, such as migraine, but a lightning strike is the only explanation that can also account for his fellow travelers also seeing a light, hearing a noise, and falling to the ground:

> On one of these journeys I was going to Damascus… About noon…as I was on the road, I saw a light from heaven, brighter than the sun, blazing around me and my companions. We all fell to the ground, and I heard a voice saying to me in Aramaic,[a] 'Saul, Saul, why do you persecute me?[199]

Paul added:

> Now those who were with me saw the light but did not understand the voice of the one who was speaking to me.[200]

Paul, now blind, was led by the hand to Damascus.

> Then the Lord said to him, 'Arise and go into the city, and you will be told what you must do.' And the men who journeyed with him stood speechless, hearing a voice but seeing no one. Then Saul arose from the ground, and when his eyes were opened he saw no one. But they led him by the hand and brought him into Damascus. And he was three days without sight, and neither ate nor drank.[201]

After 3 days of fasting, he heard a spirit telling him that a man named Ananias could heal him. Ananias heard about Paul from the Lord and traveled to the house where Paul was staying.

> Now there was a disciple in Damascus named Ananias; and the Lord said to him in a vision, 'Ananias.' And he said, 'Here I am, Lord.' And the Lord said to him, 'Get

---

198 Bullock 1994.

199 Acts 26:12-14.

200 Acts 22:9.

201 Acts 9:6-9.

> up and go to the street called Straight, and inquire at the house of Judas for a man
> from Tarsus named Saul, for he is praying, and he has seen in a vision a man named
> Ananias come in and lay his hands on him, so that he might regain his sight.'[202]

Ananias laid his hands on Paul, at which point the vision of Paul was restored:

> So Ananias departed and entered the house, and after laying his hands on him said,
> 'Brother Saul, the Lord Jesus, who appeared to you on the road by which you were
> coming, has sent me so that you may regain your sight and be filled with the Holy
> Spirit.' And immediately something like fish scales fell from his eyes, and he regained
> his sight, and he got up and was baptized; and he took food and was strengthened.[203]

Saint Paul continued to have some degree of vision and to be able to write letters. Paul wrote: "See with what large letters I am writing to you with my own hand."[204]

What ophthalmic ailment afflicted Saint Paul? One hypothesis is that lightning caused corneal epithelial opacity, which was eliminated when rubbing the eyes caused the epithelium to slough off. This type of epithelial sloughing has been demonstrated in one case following a thermal burn.[205] The problem with this hypothesis is that this type of injury is uncommon and has not actually been reported after lightning strike.

An alternative explanation is that Saint Paul experienced cataracts following the lightning strike. Cataracts after lightning strike typically occur in a delayed manner,[206] but there are exceptions, in which cataracts can occur immediately.[207] Moreover, the 3-day period of blindness preceding the cure might relate more to the period of preoperative regimen, rather than a historical account of the total period of blindness. If Saint Paul had a high myopia before his injury, then reasonable vision could have followed, even without corrective lenses.

## Three Days of Preoperative Fasting (34 CE)

Saint Paul fasted for 3 days before his ophthalmic healing. Is there any correlation with this practice in the medical literature? According to Celsus, the patient having cataract surgery would reduce intake for 3 days preoperatively.[208] Similarly, the 6th-century *Sapientia Artis Medicinae* recommended to purge the stomach of a cataract patient preoperatively with a cathartic and to bleed the patient on the

---

202 Acts 9:10-12.
203 Acts 9:17-19.
204 Galatians 6:11. Bullock 1994.
205 Bullock 1994.
206 Bullock 1994.
207 Reddy 1999.
208 Celsus, Spencer 1938.

third day.[209] Even in faraway medieval China, the cataract surgery patient was instructed in the 12th-century Nagarjuna's Comprehensive Treatise: "...take clean vegetarian diet for three days before needling."[210]

# Emperor Vespasian (69 CE)

During the siege of Jerusalem in the First Jewish–Roman War (66-73 CE), the Romans were led in battle by General Vespasian. While there, Vespasian was said to have tried to summon from Egypt the philosopher and ophthalmic healer Apollonius, who refused to travel to Judaea. Therefore, Vespasian traveled to Alexandria to meet Apollonius in a temple.[211] When Vespasian said "Make me emperor," Apollonius replied "I already have."[212]

Independent accounts reveal that Vespasian's elevation as emperor was signaled by several healings he performed while at the Temple of Serapis in Alexandria in 69 CE. One of these miracles, the healing of a blind man by applying spittle to his eyes, was described by the historian Suetonius (c. 69-after 122 CE):

> ...he [Vespasian] himself, in the meantime, passed over to Alexandria, to obtain possession of the key of Egypt. Here having entered alone, without attendants, the temple of Serapis...A poor man who was blind, and another who was lame, came both together before him, when he was seated on the tribunal, imploring him to heal them, and saying that they were admonished in a dream by the god Serapis to seek his aid, who assured them that he would restore sight to the one by anointing his eyes with his spittle, and give strength to the leg of the other, if he vouchsafed but to touch it with his heel...he [Vespasian] made the attempt publicly...and it was crowned with success in both cases.[213]

In the account of the historian Tacitus (c. 56-c. 120 CE), in addition to the blind patient, there was a man with a withered hand (rather than paralysis) who was healed by Vespasian:

> One of the common people of Alexandria, well known for his loss of sight, threw himself before Vespasian's knees, praying him with groans to cure his blindness, being so directed by the god Serapis, whom this most superstitious of nations worships before all others; and he besought the emperor to deign to moisten his cheeks and eyes with his spittle. Another, whose hand was useless, prompted by the same god, begged Caesar [Vespasian] to step and trample on it. Vespasian...directed the

---

209  Wallis 2010, p. 20.
210  Deshpande, Fan 2012, "Restoring the Dragon's Vision" p. 139. Treatise name *Longmu zang lun*.
211  Jackson 1986.
212  Jackson 1986.
213  Suetonius, Thompson 1889.

> physicians to give their opinion as to whether such blindness and infirmity could be overcome by human aid. Their reply treated the two cases differently: they said that in the first the power of sight had not been completely eaten away and it would return if the obstacles were removed; in the other, the joints had slipped and become displaced, but they could be restored if a healing pressure were applied to them… So Vespasian…did as he was asked to do. The hand was instantly restored to use, and the day again shone for the blind man.[214]

It is interesting that Tacitus presents Vespasian as consulting the Alexandrian doctors to determine whether the attempted ophthalmic healing is reasonable.

## Prognosis of Residual Vision (50-69 CE)

The Alexandrian doctors consulted by Emperor Vespasian were echoing ancient medical thought. As early as the treatise of Celsus, and today, we recognize that if a patient has some residual vision (light perception or hand motion) preoperatively, cataract surgery is more likely to succeed than if the patient has no light perception.[215] Paul of Aegina agreed that cataract patients have some residual vision, in contrast with those with have amaurosis or glaucoma, who have no light perception.[216] Ibn Isa instructed the ophthalmologist to determine "whether he can perceive sunlight and candle light. If he does, the cataract may be couched."[217] Ammar of Cairo agreed with this teaching.[218]

This teaching was not found in the Ayurvedic works attributed to Suśruta and Vāgbhata. In fact, the *Aṣṭāṅgasaṃgraha* attributed to Vāgbhata advised that cataract surgery should not be performed when blindness is "incomplete."[219] The charitable interpretation is that in antiquity, vision loss should be quite severe to justify the risks of surgery.

## The Gospel of Mark: The Blind Man at Bethsaida (70 CE)

The Gospels describe Jesus of Nazareth healing the blind. All four gospels explicitly cite the book of Isaiah in which it is prophesized that the Messiah will heal the blind. Most scholars believe that the first of the synoptic gospels to be recorded in writing was the Gospel of Mark in about 70 CE, which records Jesus healing two

---

214  Cotter 2012, pp. 40-41.

215  Celsus, Spencer 1938. "For there is hope…if at the side there persists some sensation to a flash of light."

216  Paulus Aegineta, Adams 1846, vol. 2, p. 279.

217  Ibn Isa, Wood 1936, p. 180.

218  Blodi et al. 1993, p. 149.

219  Vagbhata, Murthy 2000, vol. 3, p. 148. Chapter 17.

blind men on separate occasions. Some scholars have wondered if Jesus could have learned the art of healing the blind, including cataract surgery, during his "lost years." We only know the story of Jesus during his childhood until the age of about 12 years and then during his ministry around the age of 30 years. Cataract surgery was performed in major population centers, such as Egypt. Indeed, when Jesus was a baby, Jesus' family briefly escaped to Egypt to avoid persecution by the Roman governor Herod, according to the Gospel of Matthew.

However, ophthalmology was a specialized field. If Jesus were a trained cataract surgeon, we might have expected him to hit the ground running by performing numerous ophthalmic healings early in his ministry, and for these ophthalmic healings to occur out of proportion to the other types of healings prophesized in Isaiah.

In fact, we do not know of specific instances of Jesus healing the blind until well into his healing ministry in all the gospels. In the Gospels of Matthew and Luke, as written, there is no mention that Jesus has healed the blind until after the Sermon on the Mount. As described in the Gospel of Mark, Jesus did not heal the blind until close to the end of his ministry, when Jesus predicts his death.[220]

Moreover, blindness was not cured out of proportion to other types of healing prophesized in Isaiah. Healing the blind in the synoptic gospels is almost always paired with healings of the deaf, the mute, or the lame.

According to the Gospel of Mark, Jesus healed first a deaf-mute man and then a blind man (at Bethsaida). These two healings were obviously paired because Jesus touched and applied spittle to the affected organs (ears and tongue and then the eye) of both patients. These are the only instances in all of the synoptic gospels when Jesus uses spittle in a therapeutic manner. Recent scholarship has posited that the gospel author wanted to emphasize that Jesus was superior to the secular Roman leader Vespasian, who also healed the blind with his spittle.[221] The healing of the blind man at Bethsaida was recounted as follows:

> And they come unto Bethsaida. And they bring to him a blind man, and beseech him to touch him. And he took hold of the blind man by the hand, and brought him out of the village; and when he had spit on his eyes, and laid his hands upon him, he asked him, Seest thou aught? And he looked up, and said, I see men; for I behold them as trees, walking. Then again he laid his hands upon his eyes; and he looked steadfastly, and was restored, and saw all things clearly.[222]

---

220  Mt 16:21-23; Mk 8:31-33; Lk 9:21-22.

221  Kimondo 2011.

222  Mark 8:22-26. One distinctive aspect of these two healings of the deaf (Mk 7:32-36) and the blind man at Bethsaida (Mk 8:22-26) is that they occur in a portion of the book in which Jesus is attempting to keep his healings a secret by performing them away from the crowds of onlookers. Jesus' final instruction for the blind man at Bethsaida to avoid the village is interpreted as a request for the man to avoid telling others that he was healed. According to all three synoptic gospels, these healings occur during a later period in which Jesus attempts to

## The Healing Touch (70 CE)

In the Gospels, ophthalmic and otolaryngologic healings involved Jesus reaching out to touch the patient. When the ailment involved a demon, Jesus never touched the patient (0 of 5 healings). Of remaining healings, Jesus touched the affected part of the patient in all four ophthalmic healings (3 of 3 such healings if Matthew and Mark's first cases are identical), both otolaryngologic healings, and 4 of 12 remaining healings, related to paralysis, fever, or resurrection from the dead. Some of the nonophthalmic healings were performed just by Jesus speaking to the patient from a distance, by the patient touching Jesus' garment, or even by Jesus speaking to a family member about a patient who was not present. In contrast, the ophthalmic and otolaryngologic healings involved Jesus touching the patient, at least in some of the accounts. Moreover, Jesus could not just touch the patient once, but had to touch each part of the patient that was to be healed. Thus, the eye and ear healings mirrored actual medical or surgical procedures of the period.

## Retreatments (70 CE)

Jesus had to touch the blind man at Bethsaida twice to effect the cure. Some have offered theological explanations for this, such as to show the humanity of Jesus. Regardless of the theological explanations, the story might have resonated with ancient readers because cataract couching could require more than one attempt to succeed. Without withdrawing the couching needle from the eye, the operator might raise and lower the needle multiple times, as necessary, to get the cataract to remain depressed. Moreover, if the needle had been removed, it could later be reinserted through the same puncture site.

Retreatments were described in the ophthalmic portion of the *Suśrutasaṃhitā*.[223] The ancient author Antyllus (3rd century) advised that if the cataract rises again

---

perform cures in private, and avoid publicity surrounding his activities. All three books have a section in which Jesus is asked to provide signs of his divinity, but he asks his disciples to keep the fact that he is Messiah a secret (Mark 8:29-30; Mt 16:20; Luke 9:21). Several reasons for this secrecy could be proposed (Kimondo 2011, p. 258). Jesus is coming closer to the end of his ministry, and predicts his own death. Being open about his identity could invite retribution from the authorities. Both Mark (8:11) and Matthew (16:1) have the Pharisees demanding a sign from Jesus that he is divine at equivalent points in the narrative. In the tradition of Isaiah that healing of the deaf and the blind be mentioned together, Mark has both the deaf mute (7:32) and the blind man of Bethsaida (8:22) healed close in time, straddling the Pharisees' request. By noting that Jesus avoided publicity, the gospel authors contrast his approach with that of a secular leader, like the Roman Vespasian (Kimondo 2011, p. 258). Another theory to explain the emphasis on secrecy is that Jesus is being compared to another traveler who was disguised and whose identity was a secret at the end of his own heroic journey: Odysseus (MacDonald 2000).

223 Birch, Wujastyk 2022. According to the 878 CE manuscript: "But if the humour cannot be destroyed or if it comes back, one should apply the piercing (vyadha) once again, with appropriate oils and so on."

after couching, it should be fragmented. Moreover, if retreatment is later necessary, the needle would be introduced into the same opening.[224] Ibn Isa in the 11th century advised:

> When the cataract has been pushed down and out of the visual path, wait a little to be sure that it does not return to its old position, in which case it should again be pressed backwards and downwards... If you are obliged to intervene a second time for the reclination of a recurrent cataract, enter the needle at the same point—unless an inflammatory abscess has formed. The opening does not in these cases close as quickly as in others.[225]

Ibn Sina had similar advice and made it clear that a repeat displacement of the cataract was advised even after the instrument had been removed from the eye:

> Then remove the cystotome. Be sure that the water [cataract] goes back to its first place. If it comes back, repeat the same taking up and bringing down again to be sure that it will not come back... If...the water [cataract] has returned, enter the cystotome in the same first hole, because the first hole...has not yet healed.[226]

# Blind Bartimaeus (70 CE)

All three synoptic gospels have Jesus healing a blind man at Jericho, toward the end of his ministry. The version in the Gospel of Mark is atypical for several reasons. First, the name of the blind man is provided: Bartimaeus. This is the only time a person healed by Jesus is named in the synoptic gospels. In addition, unlike most other accounts of healing of the blind in the gospels, Jesus merely speaks to Bartimaeus and does not touch his eyes.[227]

---

224 Hirschberg 1985, vol. 2, pp. 214-216. From the Latin *Continens*.

225 Ibn Isa, Wood 1936, pp. 185-187.

226 Ibn Sina, Sardo 2014, vol. 3, p. 274.

227 Blind healing at Jericho: Mk 10:46, Mt 20:29, Lu 18:35. In Mark 10:46: "Then they came to Jericho. As Jesus and his disciples, together with a large crowd, were leaving the city, a blind man, Bartimaeus (which means 'son of Timaeus'), was sitting by the roadside begging. When he heard that it was Jesus of Nazareth, he began to shout, 'Jesus, Son of David, have mercy on me!' Many rebuked him and told him to be quiet, but he shouted all the more, 'Son of David, have mercy on me!' Jesus stopped and said, 'Call him.' So they called to the blind man, 'Cheer up! On your feet! He's calling you.' Throwing his cloak aside, he jumped to his feet and came to Jesus. 'What do you want me to do for you?' Jesus asked him. The blind man said, 'Rabbi, I want to see.' 'Go,' said Jesus, 'your faith has healed you.' Immediately he received his sight and followed Jesus along the road." So, this is a different type of ophthalmic healing story. Various reasons for this have been offered. One explanation proposed by scholars is that Bartimaeus provided a first-hand account. It has also been noted that Plato's *Timaeus* was a discourse which touched on theories of vision. In addition, the account near Jericho is a hybrid between a healing story and a "call story," in which a disciple is called to follow Jesus (Menken 2005). A final explanation is that Bartimaeus is likened to the blind seer Tiresias in the Odyssey, in that Bartimaeus understands ("sees") that Jesus' imminent destination is his own death (MacDonald 2000).

## Pliny the Elder and the Eruption at Pompeii (79 CE)

Pliny the Elder was a Roman author who died in 79 CE with the eruption of Mount Vesuvius, which destroyed the city of Pompeii. Several approaches to cataract surgery can be documented by this year, even if they may have initially begun well before the Common Era. The couching needles buried at Pompeii in 79 CE provide the earliest dated examples of these surgical implements.

## The Thorn and the Goat's Eye (79 CE)

Although we began the discussion with the Bronze Age, it is possible to perform cataract surgery using a Stone Age tool: a thorn. Early surgical tools included thorns. For instance, thorns were used by the Nahuatl in Mesoamerica to lift pterygia.[228] Thorns also frequently caused eye injuries throughout the world. When one has poor vision, accidentally impaling one's eye on a thorn might be more common. Thus, using a thorn for cataract couching could have arisen either by accident or as an outgrowth of other ophthalmic surgeries by a particularly aggressive healer.

Indeed, surgeon Robert Elliot, who worked in Madras at the turn of the 20th century, heard reports that "the long needle-like thorn of the babul-tree" was used to perform couching.[229] Other names for this tree are *Vachellia nilotica*, gum arabic tree, Egyptian or thorny acacia, and *Acacia arabica* (Fig. 10).[230] Likewise, the use of a thorn for couching has been reported in Nigeria[231] and in Sudan, the latter specifically from the *A. arabica* tree.[232]

There are hints that a thorn might have been used for cataract couching in antiquity. As noted earlier, four authors who drew on Alexandrian traditions told the story of a goat couching a cataract in its eye by running into a thorn.[233] This might seem to be just a curious story, but we must remember that very few accounts of cataract surgery from Greco-Roman antiquity have survived. The fact that this story was related by a significant fraction of all the Greco-Roman authors mentioning cataract surgery meant that the story must have enjoyed widespread circulation. This popular story may have served as a teaching tool. Just as the lightest eye was termed *glaukos*, whether in health or disease, the eye of intermediate brightness was called the goat's eye by the Greeks, again regardless of whether the eye was healthy or diseased.[234] Goats' eyes are often colored yellow or amber and are thus

---

228 Leffler et al. 2017.

229 Elliot 1918, p. 14.

230 Heuzé et al. 2016.

231 Ebeigbe 2013.

232 Al Safi 2006, pp. 156-395; Beiram 1971.

233 Leffler, Schwartz, Peterson, et al. 2018.

234 Leffler, Schwartz, Peterson, et al. 2018.

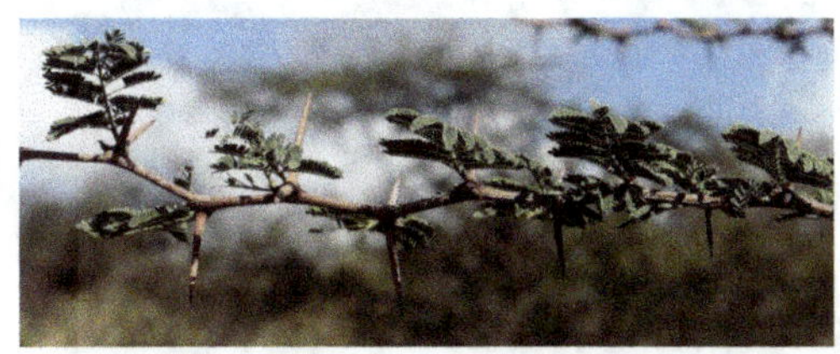

**Fig. 10.** Thorns of *Acacia nilotica*, also known as *Vachellia nilotica*, gum Arabic tree, Egyptian acacia, or thorny acacia.

intermediate in color. A cataract seen through an undilated pupil would brighten the eye a little bit, but not enough to be in the brightest category (*glaukos*). Any student would have to remember that couching worked best for the goat's eye. And given the traditional healing practices which survived for millennia in India and Africa, the procedure might really have been done with a thorn. The comparison of a surgical knife to a thorn by the medieval oculist Khalifah al-Halabi of 13th-century Aleppo might have echoed earlier surgical practices.

Several examples establish that healthy eyes of intermediate "brightness" were termed *charopos* (χαροπος), or compared with the eye of a goat. In the 4th century before the Common Era, Aristotle noted:[235]

> The eyes of human beings show great variety of colour; some are γλαυκοί [*glaukoi*] some χαροποί [*charopoi*, amber], some μελανόφθαλμοι [*melanopthalmoi*, dark], others αἰγωποί [*aigopoi*, goat-eyed, yellow].

Here, *glaukoi* was the lightest color, and *melophthalmoi* the darkest. The intermediate colors *charopoi* and the goat's eye were probably similar.

By the time of Galen, the two intermediate eye colors of Aristotle (*charopos* and the goat's eye) may have been united. Pseudo-Galen wrote that the cornea is

> ...thin in the neighbourhood of the iris, [and therefore] it lets through the underlying colour, according to whether it is μέλας [*melas*] or γλαυκότερος [*glaukoteros*] or χαροπός [*charopos*].[236]

Galen himself wrote of the differences between people:

---

235 De Generatione Animalium 5.1 (779a.35). In: Maxwell-Stuart 1981, vol. 1, p. 27; Aristotle, Taylor 1808, p. 421; Aristotle, Peck 1943, pp. 492-495.

236 Pseudo-Galen, *Medicus*, section 11. Galen, Kuhn vol. 14, p. 712. From Maxwell-Stuart 1981, vol. 1, p. 52.

> One is γλαυκός [*glaukos*], another χαροπός [*charopos*], or μέλας [melas], or whatever his eyes may be.[237]

Elsewhere, Galen again described three eye colors and wrote about the intermediate shade:

> Many people are in the habit of calling eyes of this colour 'goats' eyes.[238]

Similarly, Claudius Aelianus (c. 175-c. 235 CE) wrote about: "the wild goats of Libya": "their eyes are yellow [χαροποί, *charopoi*]".[239]

Just as the lightest color term, *glaukos*, applied to both healthy and diseased eyes, the term "goat's eye" could also be used broadly, not just for healthy eyes but also for those with disease. Here, we would expect an eye with a smaller white media opacity, such as a small corneal scar, or a white cataract seen through an undilated pupil, to produce an intermediate brightness. Hippocrates wrote in *Prorrheticon 2*:

> Pupils [κόραι, *korai*] that become grey [γλαυκούμεναι, *glaukoumenai*], silvery [ἀργυροειδέες, *argyroidees*], or blue [κυάνεαι, *kuaneai*] do not function. Slightly better than these are pupils that appear either smaller or wider than normal, or to have angles, whether…the result of a manifest cause or spontaneously. Mistinesses, clouds and specks [αἰγίδες, *aigides*] become thinner and disappear, unless some other injury occurs…or the person happens to have an earlier scar in the part, or a pterygium.[240]

Here, a small media opacity is termed *aigides*, a derivate of the Greek word for goat. Similarly, a Hippocratic author wrote in *Coan Prenotions*:

> also bad is for the eyes…to have a thin speck [αἰγίδα, *aigida*].[241]

*Aigida* has been translated in other contexts as goatskin,[242] aegis,[243] or shield,[244] from the tradition that the Gods Zeus and Athena carried a goatskin as a shield.[245]

---

237 *In Hippocrates de medici officina, Commentarius*, section 1.4. Galen, Kuhn vol 18(2), p. 664. In Maxwell-Stuart 1981, vol. 1, p. 52.

238 Galen et al. 2010, p. 31.

239 Aelian, Scholfield 1959, vol. III, pp. 158-159. Also in Maxwell-Stuart 1981, vol. 2, pp. 4-5.

240 Prorrheticon 2.20-Littré 9.48. This translation from Hippocrates, Potter 1995, Vol. VIII, pp. 260-261. Sentence with *glaukoumenai* also in Maxwell-Stuart 1981, vol. 1, p. 57; And in Magnus, Waugh 1998, part 1, p. 95.

241 Hippocrates, Potter Vol. IX. Coan Prenotions (214), 2010, pp. 154-155.

242 Strabo, Jones 2015, pp. 126-127.

243 Paton, The Greek Anthology. Vol. 1. Books 1-5. 2014, pp. 100-101.

244 Lucian 2015, pp. 264-265.

245 αἰγίς in Liddell 1940.

Hippocrates' description of a corneal speck as a goat's eye survived in medical terminology through the 19th century.[246]

Any teacher would have to explain that couching was not needed in the healthy Greek *melanos* eye, would be unsuccessful in the bright *glaukos* eye, but would work well for the intermediate eye color (the goat's eye). And the student would of course wonder how one could know the procedure worked in a goat's eye. The myth of the goat curing its own cataract could serve as a teaching tool. Pliny the Elder did tell a myth of a goat puncturing its eye to relieve suffusions:

> A she-goat cures its eyes when bloodshot [*oculos suffusos*] by pricking them on a rush, he-goats on a bramble.[247]

The Latin term for suffusion is ambiguous and was used to represent both blood and the putative humor that formed cataracts in the eye. In later authors' work, the goat was clearly curing its own cataract by puncturing its eye. One example is the account of pseudo-Galen that we reviewed earlier.[248] Similarly, Aelianus wrote:[249]

> The Goat...is...skilful at curing that mist of the eyes which doctors call 'cataract,' [ὑπόχυσιν, *hypochysin*]...men have learnt this cure from the Goat...When the Goat perceives that its sight has become clouded it goes to a bramble and applies its eye to a thorn. The thorn pricks it [ἐκέντησε, *ekentese*] and the fluid is discharged...and the Goat regains its sight...

Also, Leonidas of Alexandria wrote:[250]

> A she-goat rushing to browse on a wild pear recovered her sight from the tree, and lo! was no longer blind in one eye. For the sharp thorn pricked [ἐκέντρισεν, *ekentrisen*] the one eye. See how a tree benefited more than the surgeon's skill.

## Copper Needles (Rods) (79 CE)

Cataract surgery instruments provide an opportunity to correlate the texts with archaeological finds. The earliest materials for the couching needle specified in the Indo-Greek works are copper and bronze. As noted earlier, the code of Hammurabi

---

246  Dunglison 1846, p. 25. Incidentally, the shield ulcer of vernal keratoconjunctivitis appears to be an unrelated modern coinage, from a corneal opacity with a flat superior border, and sloping sides ending in a point inferiorly (Grayson 1969, pp. 277-279). The classic "heater-shaped shield" was first used in the Middle Ages (Boutell 1914, pp. 35-37), and therefore would not have been recognized as the shape of a shield by Hippocrates.

247  Pliny, Rackham 1940, pp. 140-141.

248  Jouanna, Allies 2012, p. 16. Sometimes written *Introductio Seu Medicus*. Galen, Kuhn vol. 14, pp. 674-676.

249  Aelian, Scholfield 1959, vol. II, pp. 120-121.

250  Paton 1917, pp. 64-65.

mentioned a bronze instrument to be used around the eye. Paulus Aegineta mentioned that the couching needle was made of copper.[251] Archaeological finds have revealed bronze couching needles at sites along the Mediterranean. The best dated are the cataract needles buried at Pompeii, with the volcanic explosion of 79 CE. Some of the instrument tips have broken off (Table 1). Cataract needles from Roman antiquity made at least partially from bronze have also been found at Maaseik and Wancennes in Belgium; Reims and Montbellet in France; Gandul in Spain; Italy; the island of Milos in Greece; and Southwest Asia Minor (Fig. 11) (Table 1). In the British Isles, ancient copper alloy cataract needles have been found at Piddington,

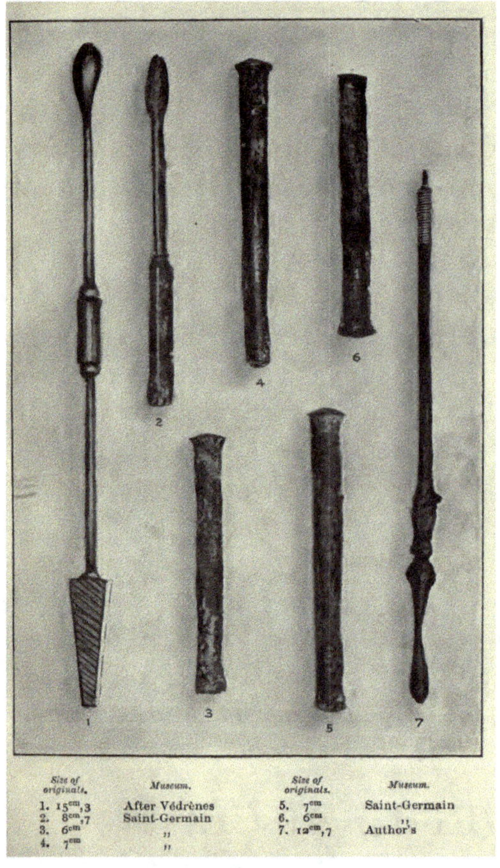

**Fig. 11.** Roman ophthalmic instruments. Item 1: Rasping specillum for curetting granular lids from trachoma. Known as *blepharoxyston* in Paulus Aegineta (III.xxii) and specillum asperatum in Celsus (VI.vi). Found in Herculaneum. Olivary point at one end and plate with transverse ridges at the other. 15.3 cm. At the Orfila Museum. Items 2-6: Instruments of the oculist Gaius Firmius Severus of the end of the 3rd century, discovered at Rheims in 1854. Handles for needles in bronze. The steel needles, which were originally attached, have disappeared. Item 2 features an olivary enlargement, which, according to Paulus, could be used to measure distance from the limbus to perforate sclera. Held at the Museum of Saint Germain-en-Laye. Instruments from this find had silver inlay. Item 7: 12.7 cm. Couching needle found at a Roman camp in Bedfordshire. Contains screw thread for a cover to protect the needle. Collection of Milne.

---

251 Paulus, Adams 1846, vol. 2, p. 280.

Caerleon in South Wales, and Carlisle auxiliary fort.[252] A bronze remnant of a cataract needle found at Palmyra (Syria) is thought to date from the late Byzantine or early Islamic periods (Table 1). Copper continued to be the first choice for couching instruments in the works of Ṣalāḥ al-Dīn al-Kaḥḥāl of 13th-century Syria.[253] Likewise, in the *Suśrutasaṃhitā*, copper was the primary material specified for couching instruments.

**Table 1. Cataract Surgery Instruments from Continental Europe and the Mediterranean.**

| Date | Where found | Comment |
| --- | --- | --- |
| 1st or early 2nd century CE | Said to be from Italy | Cataract needle, complete. Copper alloy. Olivary probe on other end, and spirally cut stem. Length 14.2 cm. Purchased by British Museum in 1968 from an antiquities dealer (Jackson 1986, item no. 23) |
| c. 200 CE | Shipwreck 3 km from Syracuse off Sicily | Remnants of an iron cataract needle, combined with a bronze scalpel. Both functional ends broken off. Length of handle 3.7 cm. Excavated 1983-1987 (Gibbins 1988; Gibbins 1989, figs. 8, 9; item PL85/128) |
| c. 50-150 CE | From a necropolis of incineration burials at La Cañada (Gandul, Sevilla) | Bronze handle with functional end of needle missing. Length 8.6 cm. Excavated 1908-1910 by George E. Bonsor (Hibbs 2018, fig. 2, item 7) |
| 79 CE | Pompeii | Bronze-handled needle, olivary terminal at one end. Found with skeletons in the Palaestra. Length 7.3 cm. Length of needle distal to ridges 1.5 cm. (Lengths based on listing of scale in Künzl 1983 as 1:1. Künzl 1983, p. 14, fig. 4, item 5, 2nd from right; Jackson 1986; Hibbs 2018). This instrument set also held: 1) two bronze instruments with olivary terminal at one end and other end (which could have been a needle or probe) broken off (Künzl 1983, p. 13, fig. 3, items 5,6); and: 2) a bronze handle with both ends broken off, which could have been needles or pointed cautery (Künzl 1983, p. 14, fig. 4, item 6). Discussion: Künzl 1983, pp. 12-15. |
| 79 CE | Pompeii | Naples, Mus. Naz., Inv. no. 116444A, found in a cylindrical probe box with six other probes and needles (Jackson 1986) |
| 79 CE | Pompeii | Pompeii Antiquarium, Inv. no. 10123, from Pompeii, Region II, Insula II, "vicino al tempieto," 1953 (Jackson 1986) |
| c. 27 BCE-150 CE ("early imperial period") | Milos, island in Greek region of Achaea | Cataract needle, bronze. Olivary terminal at other end. Athens national museum. Length 15 cm. Length of needle distal to wider ridges 3.4 cm. (Künzl 1983, pp. 40-41, fig. 10, item 4; Jackson 1986; Hibbs 2018; Milne 1907, p. 176. Hassel-Künzl 1980, p. 413) |

---

252 Leffler et al. 2021.

253 Blodi et al. 1993, p. 292.

| Date | Where found | Comment |
|---|---|---|
| Roman antiquity | Odessos (Varna, Bulgaria) | Cataract needle, with a stylus-like shape and a spherical thickening behind the tip. From the imperial tombs of Odessos. Might have been associated with a doctor. (Hassel and Künzl 1980; Tontchéva 1961, pp. 39-40, plate X, figs. 58 and 60; Meyer-Steineg 1912, tables 8, 10). Künzl (1983, p. 114) believes the illustration is too imprecise to be sure of its function. |
| Hellenistic-Roman | Island of Cos | Silver cataract needle. Globular thickening near tip, perhaps to prevent excessive insertion. Acquired by Meyer-Steineg in Cos, early 1900s. (Meyer-Steineg 1912, p. 45, plate VIII, item 10; Hassel and Künzl 1980) |
| 3rd century CE | Southwest Asia Minor | Cataract needle, made of silver. Length 13 cm. Doctor's burial site from Southwest Asia Minor. At the Romisch-Germanischen Zentralmuseums in Mainz. (Hassel and Künzl 1980, plate II, item 4) |
| 3rd century CE | Southwest Asia Minor | Cataract needle (according to Jackson 1986). In bronze. Length 16.2 cm. Other end has a second needle, with tiny spatula-like expansion near the tip. Stem design modelled after club of Hercules. May also have been for cautery or other fine procedures. Doctor's burial site from Southwest Asia Minor. At the Romisch-Germanischen Zentralmuseums in Mainz. (Hassel and Künzl 1980, plate III, item 10) |
| Period of Roman Gaul | Reims, France | A needle handle, and eight round needle handles. Bronze. Considered possibly for cataract surgery (Baker 2011, item 41). Reims. Burial site of oculist Gaius Firmius Severus. Four round handles, with a small round hole for a needle (nos. 32-35, Length 6-7.2 cm). Four handles with an angular cross section, for insertion of a needle, nos. 34-38 additionally as a scalpel handle (nos. 36-39, Length 4 to 6.2 cm). Musée des Antiquités Nationales in Saint-Germain-en-Laye. Voinot 1999 catalog #104. Item numbering above as per Künzl 1983, pp. 61-67, fig. 37, nos. 32-39. Discussed by Milne 1907, pp. 21, 69-70, table 2, 1-5.7; 16,2-6; 20,3-4;21,2.4; 23,2.4; 29,2. And Hassel-Künzl 1980, p. 415 |
| Period of Roman Gaul | River Saône, Montbellet (Saône-et-Loire) | Five cataract needles, two of which are hollow. (Feugère et al. 1985, pp. 24-41) |
| 50 BCE-476 CE | River Maas, Maaseik (Limburg), Belgium | Bronze needle, with tip broken off. Might be a cataract needle (Baker 2011). Length 15.6 cm. Other end is olivary. Excavated in 1968. (Heymans 1979, Figure 2, Item 5; Feugère et al. 1988:35; Heymans and Jansenns 1975-76. |
| 27 BCE-476 CE "Imperial period" | Wancennes (Namur), Belgium | Needle handle, bronze. Burial site. Considered cataract needle. Musée de la Société Archéologique. (Künzl 1983, p. 70; Baker 2011). Künzl 1983; Milne 1907, p. 21; Hassel-Künzl 1980, p. 415 |

| Date | Where found | Comment |
|---|---|---|
| Roman antiquity | In the River Tiber in Rome | Cataract needle. Provenance uncertain. At the Museo Nazionale Romano (Reggiani Massarini 1988, fig. 9; Baker 2004) |
| Probably early Islamic (7th century or later), possibly late Byzantine (pre-7th century) | Palestine or Syria | Bronze remnant of cataract needle. Length 7.5 cm. Excavated from Palmyra ruins by Russian Baron Ustinov and purchased by S. Holth in Oslo in 1918/1919. (Bliquez 1984; Holth 1919, item 23; Holth 1924) |

# Pharmacologic Mydriasis (79 CE)

Pliny the Elder wrote about pharmacologic mydriasis before paracentesis for cataracts using a plant called *anagallis*:

> The anagallis is called 'corchoron' by some…The juice…applied with honey, disperses films upon the eyes, suffusions of blood in those organs resulting from blows, and argema with a red tinge: if used in combination with Attic honey, they are still more efficacious. The anagallis has the effect also of dilating the pupil; hence the eye is anointed with it before the operation of couching for cataract.[254]

This passage has been a mystery for two reasons. First, it is not obvious that preoperative dilation would help with couching. It would help one see the needle in front of the cataract better, but it could increase the likelihood of the cataract being accidentally dislocated into the anterior chamber. Perhaps, that is the reason we only hear about preoperative pupillary dilation from Pliny, and from no other ancient or medieval author.

The second reason that this passage has been mysterious is that anagallis does not actually dilate the pupil. Magnus "made comprehensive tests with our pimpernel without being able to detect any mydriatic effect."[255] Magnus offers the possible solution to this quandary by proposing that both anagallis and sleepy strychnos can go by the name *halicacabum*.[256] However, *halicacabum* simply denotes a bad poison[257]; therefore, this overlap in terminology is not terribly specific.

---

254 Pliny et al. 1900, p. 137. Book 25, Chap. 92.

255 Magnus, Waugh 1998, vol. 1, p. 234.

256 Magnus, Waugh 1998, vol. 1, p. 234. Dioscorides et al. 2000 (IV, 73), Pliny (Book XXI, CV, 177 ff.).

257 Dioscorides et al. 2000, English translation, Section 4-27, p. 571; section 4-72, p. 619; section 4-73, p. 620; section 4-75, p. 623.

We would offer an alternative solution. Dioscorides details that both anagallis and its mixture with hyoscyamus benefited the eyes and went by the name *chelidonia*. Under the heading *anagallis*, Dioscorides reports:

> With Attic [Athenian] honey it mends *argemae* [small white ulcers on the cornea] and helps moisture of the eyes...Some call it *punicea*...others, *chelidonion*...The common *anagallis* some call *corchoros, halicacabus*,...[258]

Under the heading *Othonna*, Dioscorides reports:

> Some say othonna is the juice of *chelidonia major*...some that it is a mixture of the juices of *anagallis coerulea, hyoscyamus* and poppy, and some say that it is the juice of a certain primitive herb called *othonna*, and that it grows in the part of Arabia that lies towards Egypt...It is juiced and put into eye medicines for when there is need of cleansing the eyes; it has a biting nature and removes all things that darken the pupils whatsoever.[259]

Therefore, when Pliny reports that anagallis dilated the eyes, he might have been denoting a mixture that contained hyoscyamus as well.

# Demosthenes Philalethes (1st century)

Demosthenes Philalethes, thought to be of the Herophilean school, wrote a work *Ophthalmicus* in the 1st century CE, portions of which have survived in the 6th-century writings of Aëtius of Amida and other works.[260] Demosthenes dealt with numerous surgical conditions: staphyloma (*Stafiloma*), pterygia (*Pterigia*), chalazia (*Calaza*), lagophthalmos, eyelid abscesses, and "Paracentesis" for cataract.[261] With respect to cataract surgery, the medieval author Matthaeus Silvaticus wrote: "Paracentesis. There is a perforation which takes place in the eyes to reposition that frozen (or congealed) water, which they call a cataract, according to Demosthenes own chapter."[262] Whether the original text of Demosthenes believed "water" was the source of the cataract or whether Silvaticus was influenced by later Arabic authors in this respect is unknown. However, the passage establishes that Demosthenes wrote about cataract surgery.

There are some interesting parallels between Greek writings and chapter 7, *Uttaratantra*, of the Sushruta Samhita with respect to entoptic phenomena, diplopia

---

258 Dioscorides et al. 2000, English translation, pp. 349-351. Section 2-209.

259 Dioscorides et al. 2000, English translation, pp. 355-356, Section 2-213.

260 Von Staden 1989, pp. 69-578; Aetius, Waugh 2000.

261 Von Staden 1989, pp. 576-577; Shastid 1917, vol. 11, pp. 8680, 8683; Hirschberg 1919;

262 *"Paracentesis. Est perforatio, quae fit in oculis ad deponendam aquam illam congelatam, quam cataractam dicunt, ut Demosthenes proprio capite."* Hirschberg 1919; von Staden 1989, pp. 576-577.

from double pupils, and comparison of the lens with a lentil, as illustrated later. These parallels raise the possibility that this portion of the Sushruta Samhita was influenced by the Greek authors.

## Seeing flies, hairs, webs, circles (1st century)

Aëtius recorded entoptic phenomena associated with early cataracts:

> According to Demosthenes. Cataract is an effusion of exudate, which hardens in the pupil, so that when it has become complete, it abrogates the sight. But in the beginning of the formation of a cataract the following happens to the patients: It appears to them as if little flies and tiny dark bodies continually floated before the eyes; a few see formations resembling hairs, others things like threads of wool or spiderwebs, to others circles appear about the flames of lamps.[263]

This passage survived, with the entoptic phenomena listed in the same order (flies, hairs, webs, circles), in the Sushruta Samhita, *Uttaratantra*, Chapter VII, on diseases of the pupillary region (*dṛṣṭi*):

> Vision becomes more disturbed when *doṣa* [a fault] reaches the second layer; due to this, the patient sees (falsely) flies, mosquitos, hairs, webs, circles, banners, rays, ear-rings, various movements of stars, rains, clouds and darkness.[264]

## Double Pupils and Double Vision (1st century)

Demosthenes wrote about "*dicoriasis*", or double pupil:[265] "*Dicoriasis Demo.ē due pupille in eod ē oculo constitute...*"[266] What significance did a double pupil have to an eye surgeon in that era?

We will not find out from Pliny, who wrote that among the Triballi, the Illyrians, the Scythians, and those in Pontus there were people with double pupils ("*pupillas binas, oculo geminam pupillam*") who could injure with their glance.[267]

---

263 Shastid 1917 vol. 11, p. 8669.

264 The 1916 Bhishagratna translation stated: "False images of gnats, flies, hairs, nets or cobwebs, rings (circular patches), flags, ear-rings appear to the sight, and the external objects seem to be enveloped in mist or haze as if laid under a sheet of water or as viewed in rain and on cloudy days and meteors of different colours seem to be falling constantly in all directions..."(Sushruta, Bhishagratna 1916, vol. 3, pp. 25-26)

265 von Staden 1989, p. 577.

266 Januensis 1474 "dicoriasis".

267 Pliny, Rackham 1940, vol. 2, book VII, pp. 516-519.

A more medical explanation came from Calcidius in the 4th century CE, who offered that dicoriasis could lead to double vision (diplopia):

> They [the Geometricians, in agreement with the Peripatetics] also maintain that there is a single ray coming out of one and the other eye, invoking the condition called *hypochysis* and the vision of those who, it is believed, see double and have two pupils in each eye. Indeed, when a thick humor settles in the eyes without occupying or obstructing the entire orbit, but standing in the middle and leaving free on each side a portion of the gaze, then when the ray is broken, the gaze is divided into two and those who suffer from this disease believe they see double. Medical practice detects the same fault in the case of double pupils. Indeed, where there are two pupils, with the natural pupil objects are correctly seen, while the other one only sees images of them. This is why doctors remove that which exceeds the requirements of nature, and perform an ablation of the unnatural pupil, by surgery. When this is done, the natural integrity of vision is restored.[268]

Calcidius referred to "*hypochysis*" obscuring vision and also indicated that someone having double vision from twin pupils ("*geminis pupulis*") would have the physician remove the "unnatural pupil through surgical intervention," perhaps by placing a scar ("*cicatrice*") in front of the unwanted pupil.[269]

The Sushruta Samhita, *Uttaratantra*, Chapter VII, on diseases of the pupillary region (*dṛṣṭi*) recorded:

> If the damage is in central portion of *dṛṣṭi* he perceives single object as double.[270]

Vāgbhata also recorded that the central pupillary obstruction could produce double vision.

# Healing Baths and Pools (90 CE)

Several religious texts have the eyes or the body washed to effect an ophthalmic cure. Ananias baptized Saint Paul after curing his blindness.[271] Jesus told the congenitally blind man in the Gospel of John (chapter 9) to "wash in the pool of Siloam" to finish the cure. Similarly, John mentions a healing pool in Jerusalem, named Bethesda, where the blind would congregate to be healed (Jn 5:2-9). At this pool, Jesus healed a paralytic by simply commanding him to rise.

Was bathing the eyes or the body part of traditional ophthalmic healing? Liquids would sometimes be used to bathe the eye during or just after the procedure. A bath

---

268 Bakhouche 2013.
269 Calcidius, Magee 2016, p. 504.
270 Susruta, Sharma 2014, vol. 3, p. 140.
271 Acts 9:17-19.

was usually forbidden during the early postoperative period and, therefore, marked the completion of the patient's recovery.

In *Sapientia Artis Medicinae*, after cataract couching is performed, the patient could have a bath on postoperative day 10.[272] In the medieval treatise of Ammar of Cairo, the patient should take a bath 40 days after cataract couching.[273]

In the Ayurvedic treatises of Suśruta and Vāgbhata, the eye was sprinkled with breast milk while the couching needle was still in the eye. The works of Vāgbhata forbid the patient from bathing for 7 days after the procedure.[274]

The Chinese treatise *Longshu pusa yanlun* of the early 9th century advised after cataract surgery: "For one month after opening the patient should not wash his face. There is a fear of water entering the aperture made by the needle and it will harm the eye."[275]

# The Man Born Blind in the Gospel of John (90-110 CE)

Jesus cured a man born blind in the ninth chapter of the Gospel of John (9:1-41):

> And as he passed by, he saw a man blind from his birth. And his disciples asked him, saying, Rabbi, who sinned, this man, or his parents, that he should be born blind? Jesus answered, Neither did this man sin, nor his parents: but that the works of God should be made manifest in him...When I am in the world, I am the light of the world. When he had thus spoken, he spat on the ground, and made clay of the spittle, and anointed his eyes with the clay, and said unto him, Go, wash in the pool of Siloam (which is by interpretation, Sent). He went away therefore, and washed, and came seeing... Since the world began it was never heard that any one opened the eyes of a man born blind. If this man were not from God, he could do nothing.

The fact that the observers understood that it was unprecedented for someone to restore vision for the congenitally blind evinces a clear understanding of amblyopia in antiquity (Fig. 12). This understanding is found nowhere else in the ancient Greco-Roman secular or religious literature. Celsus' work and the Sushruta Samhita taught that cataract couching was less likely to be successful in the very young.[276] But the man born blind was no longer a child and, therefore, could have been treated according to these medical texts.

---

272 Wallis 2010, p. 20. "Administer clean salty brine to the eyes and again place egg yolk over the eyes with soft wool...on the tenth [day], let him have a bath and he will be better."

273 Blodi et al. 1993, p. 159.

274 Vagbhata, Murthy 2017, "Astanga Hrdayam," chapter 16. Vaghbata, Murthy 2000, "Astanga Samgraha," vol. 3, p. 151.

275 Deshpande, Fan 2012, "Restoring the Dragon's Vision," p. 111.

276 Leffler, Klebanov et al. 2020.

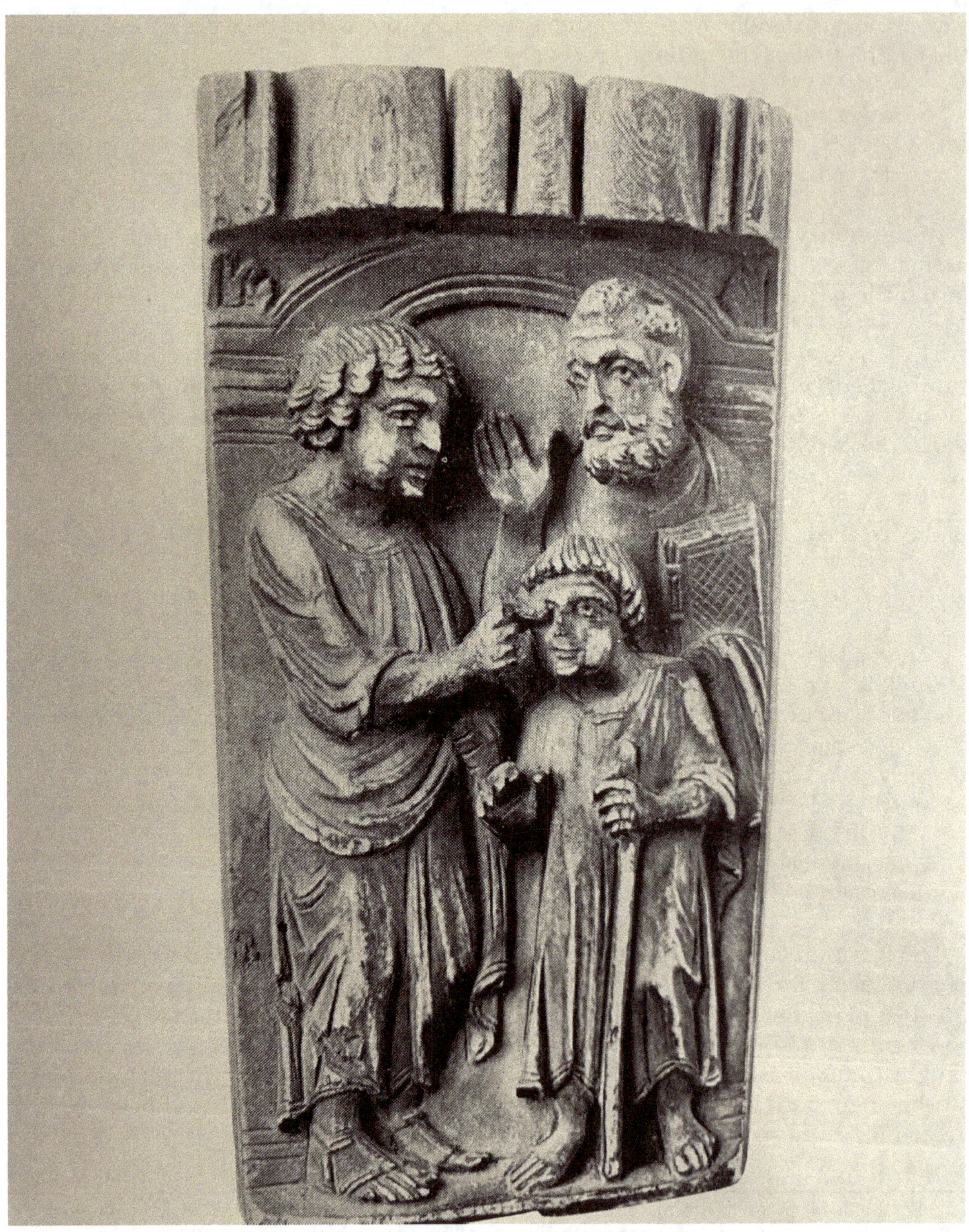

**Fig. 12.** Cure of a man born blind from a 6th-century ivory medicine box at the Vatican Library (Grisar 1907, p. 160).

As with the Gospel of John, the ancient Buddhist literature recognized the special status of the congenitally blind. The Lotus Sutra, which could date from as early as 50 CE, compares spiritual enlightenment to the cure of one born blind by a doctor. The Nirvana Sutra explicitly states that a doctor could cure blindness in general, but not if the blindness was congenital.

## Silver Instruments (100 CE)

In the Mediterranean region, ancient silver cataract instruments have been recovered (Table 1). For the hollow needles of Montbellet, dating to about 100 CE, silver was used for the inlay and to construct the internal wire.[277] A silver cataract needle with a globular thickening near the tip to prevent excessive insertion, thought to date from the Hellenistic-Roman period, was acquired by Meyer-Steineg from a local collection on the island of Cos in the early 1900s (Table 1, Figure 13). Another silver cataract needle came from a 3rd-century CE doctor's burial site in Southwest Asia Minor (Table 1). The instruments of the 3rd-century oculist Severus had silver inlay (Fig. 11) (Table 1). Silver couching needles were the preferred tools of Benevenutus Grassus in the 12th or 13th century.[278]

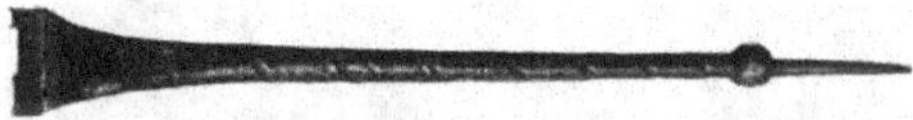

**Fig. 13.** Silver couching needle of the Hellenistic-Roman period from the island of Cos.

Silver couching instruments are described in some Ayurvedic works by the medieval period, but ancient use in India cannot be proved. Silver couching instruments do not appear in the medieval Chinese literature.

## The Lens as a Lentil (2nd century)

Lentils may have originated in the Turkey–Iraq–Syria area, but they have long been cultivated both along the Mediterranean and in India.[279] The lens was compared to a lentil because of its shape in the writings of Rufus of Ephesus (80-150 CE) and the anonymous author called pseudo-Rufus.[280] Likewise, Abu Ali al-Husain Ibn Sina (c. 980-1037 AD), known later as Avicenna, was familiar with the writings of Rufus

---

277 Feugère 1985.
278 Grapheus, Wood, 1929, p. 33.
279 Nene 2006.
280 Robinson, Lovicu 2004, p. 5; Longrigg 1988.

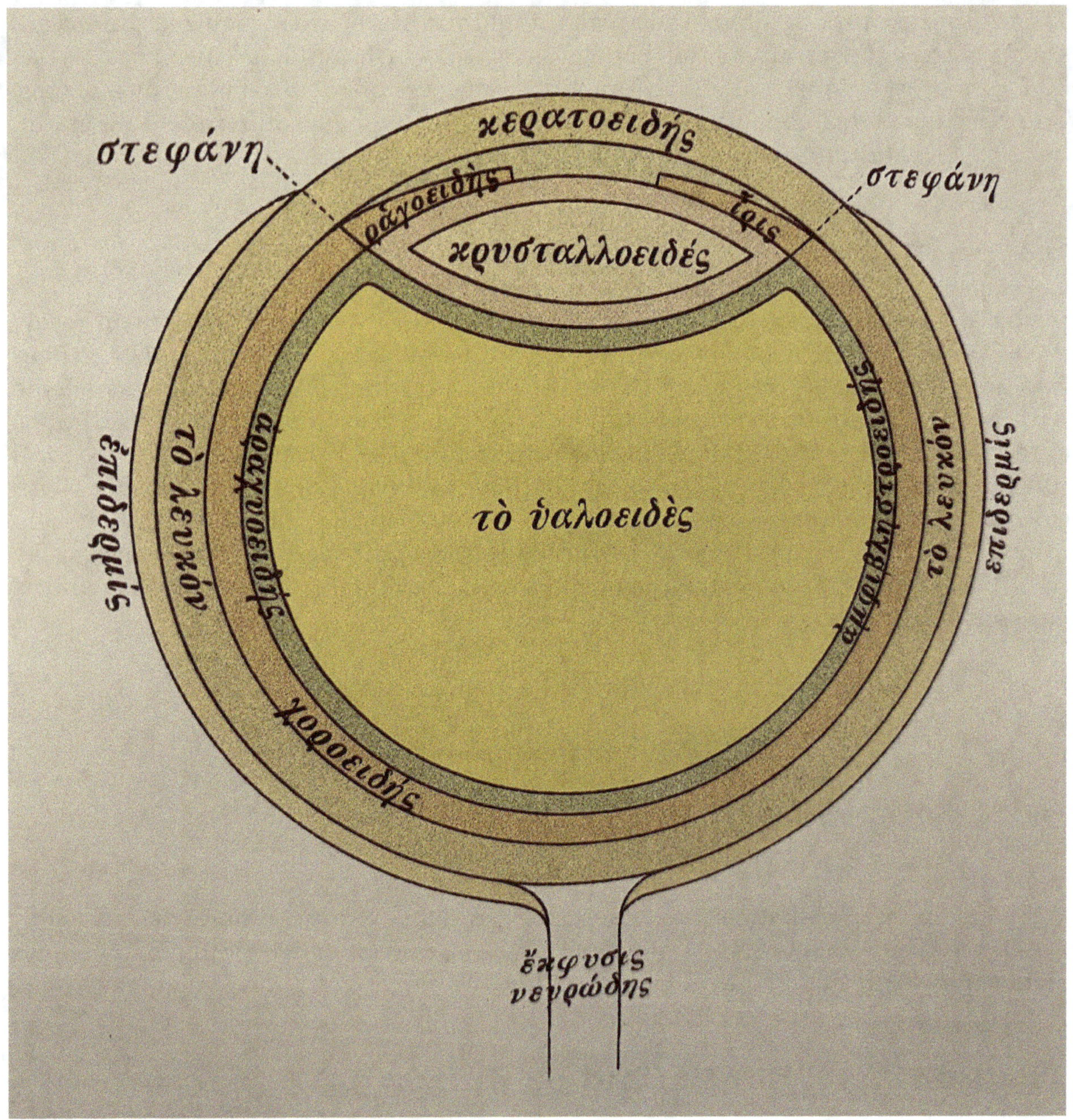


**Fig. 14.** The anatomy of the eye, with an anterior crystalline lens, according to an interpretation of the writings of Rufus of Ephesus. Rufus compared the crystalline lens to a lentil.

and also compared the lens to a lentil (Fig. 14).[281] This understanding must have resulted from dissection of the eye to examine the shape of the lens. This teaching may have spread eastward, as both Suśruta and Ugrāditya also compared the size of the pupil to a lentil, as discussed in the chapter on India.

---

281 Shastid 1913, vol. XI, p. 8580; Ibn Sina, Sardo 2014, p. 207.

## Wind Coming from the Abdomen (2nd century)

The idea that a diseased wind coming from the abdomen could cause symptoms similar to those caused by cataracts is found in both the Greek and Chinese literature. Galen wrote in the 2nd century in *On Diseases and Symptoms*:

> When certain vapours rise up from the stomach, and particularly whenever they do not digest properly, symptoms occur like those with cataracts (*hypochyma*)... Symptoms similar to this are the illusion of a cataract (*hypochyma*) occurring in the eyes in gastric conditions.[282]

Similarly, Hunain in the 11th century referred to visual loss resulting "from vapours rising from the stomach to the head."[283] Hunain believed that the visual "phantasms" resulting from stomach disorders were not true cataracts and would affect both eyes equally.[284]

In the Chinese literature, this vision-impairing wind rose from the liver, rather than the stomach. For instance, Zhao Yuanfang's 7th-century treatise *Zhu Bing Yuan Hou Lun* (*Treatise on the Causes and Symptoms of Diseases*) stated that blindness is the result of wind coming from the liver into the eyes.[285] Later, the *Treatise of Bodhisattva Nagarjuna on Eye (Diseases)* of the early 9th century, a text that covered cataract couching, stated: "This is the beginning of a disease *Que mu* (night blindness). Its chief reason is liver wind."[286]

## Iron Needles (200 CE)

The next material used to construct the couching instruments was iron (Table 1). Its use might have arisen independently in several locations. Iron cataract needles have been found in a shipwreck off the coast of Sicily from 200 CE.[287] The handles of three iron instruments, which were probably cataract needles, were excavated from a burial site at Stanway, near Colchester, UK, in 1996.[288]

Iron may have been used in the East as well. The earliest surviving manuscript of the *Suśrutasaṃhitā*, from 878 CE, advises cataract couching with "the probe (*śalākā*) made of copper or iron."[289] Iron was also listed as a secondary material for

---

282  Galen Johnston, 2006, pp. 211, 215; Kuhn VII.97-VII.106;

283  Hunain, Meyerhof 1928, p. 51.

284  Hunain, Meyerhof 1928, pp. 70-71.

285  Ka Wai Fan 2005.

286  Deshpande, Fan 2012 p. 88. Treatise name *Longshu pusa yanlun*.

287  Edge 1988; Gibbins 1989.

288  Leffler et al. 2021.

289  Susruta et al. 2021, Uttaratantra, adhyāya 16 (17 in the vulgate): 51-52, p. 37.

the couching instrument later in this manuscript: "A commendable probe should be made of silver, iron or gold (*śātakumbhī*)."[290] In the text *Aṣṭāṅgasaṃgraha*, surgical instruments can be made with tempered steel.[291] According to the Samyuktagama from the eastern Jin Dynasty (350-431 CE): "*Tathāgata* (Thus Come One) surpasses mundane physicians in ophthalmology because he understands how to cut off the cataract (*timira*) of ignorance with the iron of wisdom."[292]

## Antyllus (2nd to 4th centuries)

Antyllus is our next important Greek surgical author. Based on citations, he must have followed the early 2nd-century surgeon Archigenes and must have preceded the 4th-century author Oribasius.[293] As Mathias Witt reviews elsewhere in this volume, Antyllus is referred to as an "Alexandrian" by the Arabic authors, which could refer to his period of activity (before the Islamic conquest of Egypt), rather than just the city of Alexandria. But, as Antyllus refers to the speech patterns in Egypt and Syria, he seems to have been familiar with this general region.

With respect to cataract surgery, Antyllus seems to have heavily influenced numerous subsequent surgeons. The cataract surgical methods of Ibn Isa, Ammar, and Ibn Sina (Avicenna) have very specific and idiosyncratic elements, which derive from Antyllus. Ibn Sina (Avicenna) actually cites Antyllus, but not with respect to ophthalmology.

Antyllus' cataract method is known only from surviving Arabic works, or their Latin translations. In the 13th century, Ṣalāḥ al-Dīn al-Kaḥḥāl recorded:

> Antyllos prohibits the cataract patient to be bled by scarification or to take fish or meat of small animals or the wine of dates or vegetables; he permits them to eat only once, in the middle of the day.[294]

Most of our information on Antyllus' cataract method was preserved by Abu Bakr Muhammad Ibn Zakariya al-Rāzī (known in Latin as Rhazes, c. 865-925) in his encyclopedia *Kitab al-Hawi fi al-tibb*, known in translation as *Liber Continens* (Figs. 15, 16). Hirschberg translated some portions of Antyllus' method.

> Antilus [*Antilis*] says: 'A cataract [*Catarracta*] occurs in the eyes from the coldness of the complexion, and is brought together by the coldness of the air and the humidity of the eyes: and it is cured with perforation [*perforatione*], which is for a moderate congealing; and when it is for a strong congealing that is too subtle, it is not cured

---

290  Susruta et al. 2021, Uttaratantra, adhyāya 16 (17 in the vulgate): 67, p. 39.

291  Meulenbeld 1999, vol. 1A, p. 509.

292  Deshpande 2000. *Samyuktagama* (T 99:36:259c-260c).

293  Grant 1960, Grant 1961.

294  Blodi et al. 1993, pp. 281, 302.

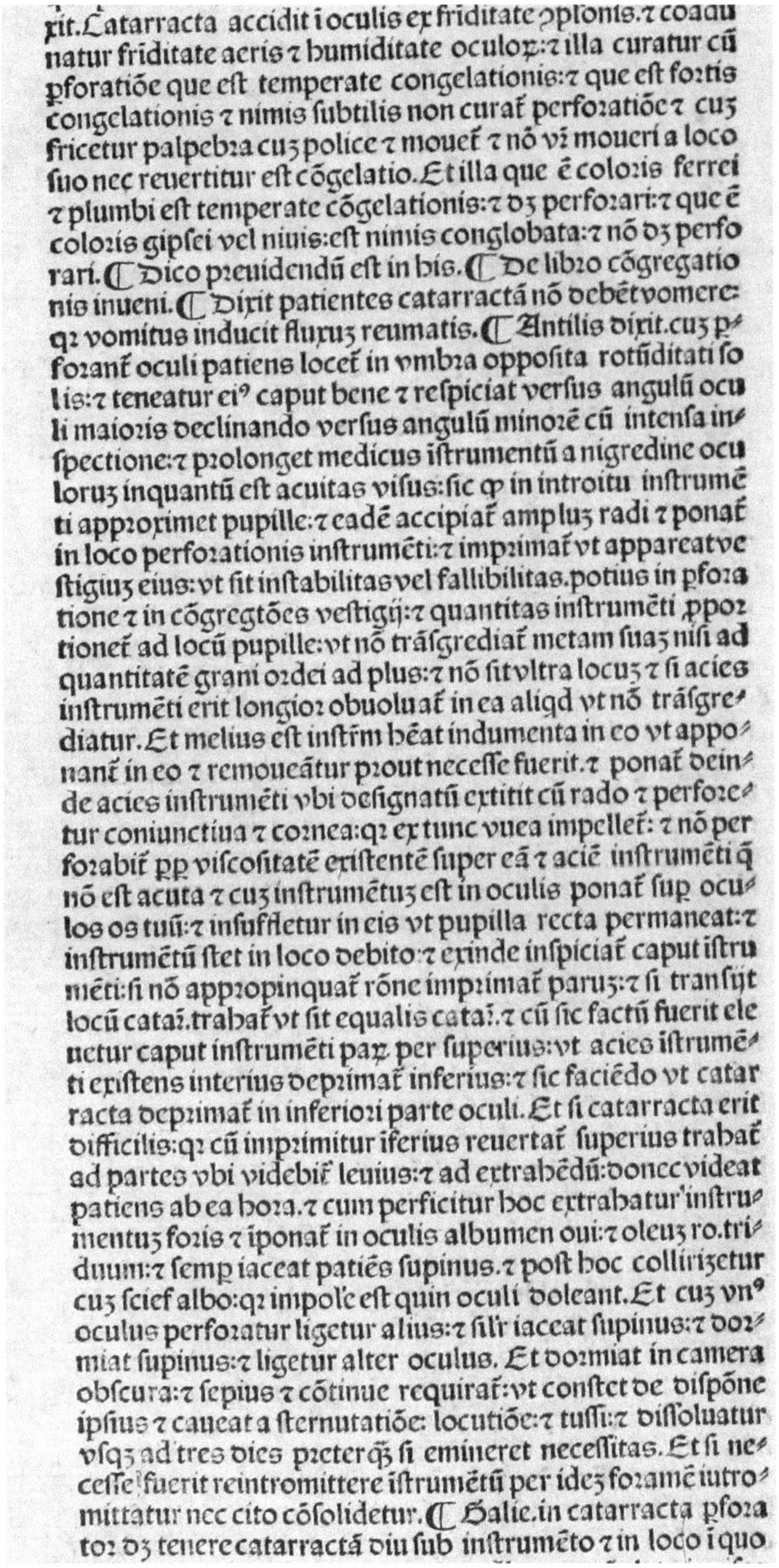

rit.Catarracta accidit i oculis ex friditate ꝓplōnis.ꞇ coaqu
natur friditate aeris ꞇ humiditate oculoꝝ:ꞇ illa curatur cū
ꝑforatiōe que est temperate congelationis:ꞇ que est foꝛtis
congelationis ꞇ nimis subtilis non curaꝛ perfoꝛatiōe ꞇ cuꝫ
fricetur palpebꝛa cuꝫ police ꞇ moueꝛ ꞇ nō vꝛ moueri a loco
suo nec reuertitur est cōgelatio.Et illa que ē coloꝛis ferrei
ꞇ plumbi est temperate cōgelationis:ꞇ oꝫ perfoꝛari:ꞇ que ē
coloꝛis gipſei vel niuis:est nimis conglobata:ꞇ nō oꝫ perfo
rari.Ⅽ Dico pꝛeuidendū est in his.Ⅽ De libꝛo cōgregatio
nis inueni.Ⅽ Diꝛit patientes catarractá nō oebét vomere:
qꝛ vomitus inducit fluꝛuꝫ reumatis.Ⅽ Antilis diꝛit.cuꝫ ꝑ
foꝛanꝛ oculi patiens loceꝛ in vmbꝛa opposita rotūditati ſo
lis:ꞇ teneatur eiꝰ caput bene ꞇ reſpiciat verſus angulū ocu
li maioꝛis oeclinando verſus angulū minoꝛé cū intenſa in
ſpectione:ꞇ pꝛolonget medicus iſtrumentū a nigredine ocu
loruꝫ inquantū est acuitas viſus:sic ꝙ in introitu inſtrumē
ti appꝛoꝛimet pupille:ꞇ eadé accipiaꝛ ampluꝫ radi ꞇ ponaꝛ
in loco perfoꝛationis instrumēti:ꞇ impꝛimaꝛ vt appareatve
ſtigiuꝫ eius:vt sit instabilitas vel fallibilitas.potius in pſoꝛa
tione ꞇ in cōgregtōes vestigij:ꞇ quantitas instrumēti ꝓpoꝛ
tioneꝛ ad locū pupille:vt nō trāſgrediaꝛ metam suaꝫ nisi ad
quantitaté grani oꝛdei ad plus:ꞇ nō sit vltra locuꝫ ꞇ si acies
instrumēti erit longioꝛ obuoluaꝛ in ea aliqd vt nō trāſgre
diatur.Et melius est inſtr̄m bēat indumenta in eo vt appo
nanꝛ in eo ꞇ remoueātur pꝛout necesse fuerit.ꞇ ponaꝛ dein
de acies instrumēti vbi oesignatū eꝛtitit cū rado ꞇ perfoꝛe
tur coniunctiua ꞇ coꝛnea:qꝛ eꝛ tunc vuea impelleꝛ:ꞇ nō per
foꝛabiꝛ ꝑꝑ viscositaté eꝛistenté super eā ꞇ acié instrumēti q̄
nō est acuta ꞇ cuꝫ instrumētuꝫ est in oculis ponaꝛ ſup ocu
los os tuū:ꞇ insuffletur in eis vt pupilla recta permaneat:ꞇ
instrumētū stet in loco oebito:ꞇ eꝛinde inſpiciaꝛ caput iſtru
méti:ſi nō appꝛopinquaꝛ rōne impꝛimaꝛ paruꝫ:ꞇ si transijt
locū cataꝛ.trahaꝛ vt sit equalis cataꝛ.ꞇ cū sic factū fuerit ele
netur caput instrumēti paꝛ. per superius:vt acies iſtrumē
ti eꝛistens interius depꝛimaꝛ inferius:ꞇ sic faciēdo vt catar
racta depꝛimaꝛ in inferioꝛi parte oculi.Et si catarracta erit
oifficilis:qꝛ cū impꝛimitur iferius reuertaꝛ superius trahaꝛ
ad partes vbi videbiꝛ lenius:ꞇ ad eꝛtrahēdū:oonec videat
patiens ab ea hoꝛa.ꞇ cum perficitur hoc eꝛtrahatur inſtru
mentuꝫ foꝛis ꞇ iponaꝛ in oculis albumen oui:ꞇ oleuꝫ ro.tri
duum:ꞇ ſemp iaceat patiēs supinus.ꞇ post hoc colliriꝫetur
cuꝫ ſcieꝛ albo:qꝛ impoſſe est quin oculi doleant.Et cuꝫ vnꝰ
oculus perfoꝛatur ligetur alius:ꞇ ſilꝛ iaceat supinus:ꞇ doꝛ
miat supinus:ꞇ ligetur alter oculus. Et doꝛmiat in camera
obſcura:ꞇ ſepius ꞇ cōtinue requiraꝛ:vt constet de oispōne
ipſius ꞇ caueat a sternutatiōe: locutiōe:ꞇ tuſſi:ꞇ oiſſoluatur
vſqꝫ ad tres dies pꝛeteꝛqꝫ ſi emineret neceſſitas.Et si ne
ceſſe fuerit reintromittere iſtrumētū per ideꝫ foꝛamē iutro
mittatur nec cito cōſolidetur.Ⅽ Halie.in catarracta pſoꝛa
toꝛ oꝫ tenere catarractā oiu ſub inſtrumēto ꞇ in loco iquo

**Fig. 15.** Cataract couching method of Antyllus from Rhazes' *Liber Continens* (Rhazes 1529, Book 2, capitulum 3, section QQ, car. 41, image 102).

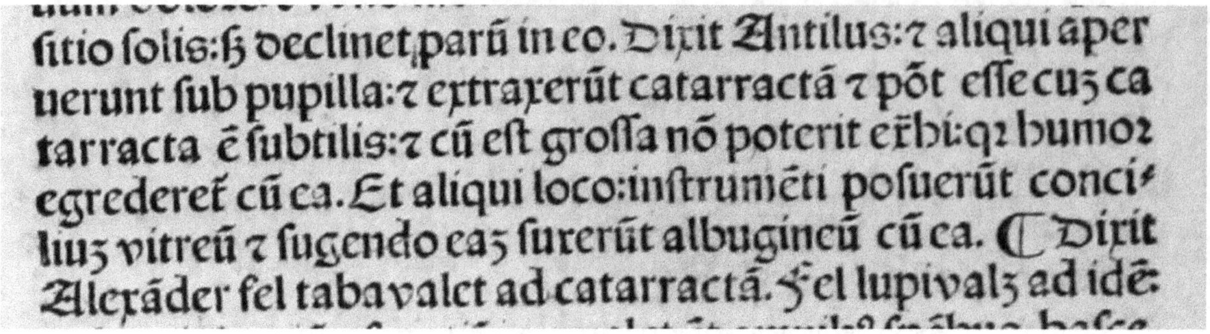

fitio folis:ß declinet parū in eo. Dixit Antilus:z aliqui aper
uerunt fub pupilla:z extraxerūt catarractá z pōt effe cuz ca
tarracta ē fubtilis:z cū eft groffa nó poterit exbi:qz humoz
egrederef cū ea. Et aliqui loco:inftruméti pofuerūt conci-
liuz vitreū z fugendo eaz furerūt albugineū cū ea. ⫶Dixit
Alexáder fel tabavalet ad catarractá. Fel lupivalz ad idē.

**Fig. 16.** Cataract extraction of Antyllus by inferior corneal incision (or by suction) from Rhazes' *Liber Continens* (Rhazes 1529, Book 2, capitulum 3, section QQ, car. 41, image 102). This passage is discussed in a subsequent chapter.

by perforation, and when the brow is rubbed with the thumb and moved, and it does not seem to move from its place nor does it return, it is a congealing. And that which is of an iron [*ferrei*] or lead [*plumbi*] colour reflects a moderate congealing: and it should be perforated: and that which is of the colour of gypsum [*gipsei*] or snow [*niuis*] is too dense: and it should not have be perforated.' I say that care should be taken in these matters. I found this in the book of congregation [*libro congregationis*]. It said that patients should not vomit: because vomit induces the flow of rheum.[295]

A second paragraph follows:

Antilis [*Antillîche*]: For the cataract operation [*qadh*] the patient is seated in a shadow and faces the sun. The head of the patient is held firmly.[296]

Order him to turn his pupil [*hadaqa*] to the side of the largest (internal) angle while looking at you; as if he wanted to make a turning movement towards the small (external) angle.[297]

---

295 Rhazes 1529, Book 2, capitulum 3, section QQ, car. 41, image 102. At our request, David Butterfield, PhD translated this paragraph.

296 Hirschberg 1982, vol. 1, p. 348. Arabic transliteration from Meyerhof (1932). Hirschberg translated the cataract method of Antyllus twice, with somewhat varied wording each time, as he was prone to resolve uncertainties by drawing parallels with other Arabic works. Here, we present the version of Hirschberg's translation in English which is closest to those of Feugère and Meyerhof, or, the translation of Feugère or Meyerhof if Hirschberg's wording appears in error.

297 Meyerhof 1932. Feugère (1985) translated this passage as "One orders the patient to move his pupil towards the greater (inner) corner of the eye, while looking at you [the doctor] as he would turn his eye to the smaller (outer) corner of the eye". Hirschberg translated this passage from the Latin Continens, folio 41V, as: "The patient should look toward the nasal canthus (the greater canthus) and keep his eye in that direction." (Hirschberg 1985, vol. 2, pp. 213-214) After 1905, Hirschberg reviewed the Arabic manuscript, and translated this sentence as: "...he is asked to look with the affected eye toward his nose; this is therefore a kind of squinting toward the nose (and a looking away from the temple)".(Hirschberg 1982, vol. 1, p. 348) This seems to be inaccurate—the greater canthus, rather than the nose, is

This instruction is difficult to interpret even in the original Arabic, but might mean that after converging the eyes, the patient looks upward toward the doctor.[298]

> Take the measurement of the distance from the dark (of the eye) according to the length of the tip of the needle [*miqdah*], so that the tip, when it fully enters the eye, reaches the pupil [*nâzir*].[299]

Ṣalāḥ al-Dīn al-Kaḥḥāl recorded:

> Antyllos says: The distance of the perforation from the limbus should be as long as the distance of the pupil from the limbus.[300]

Returning to Antyllus' method in the text of al-Rāzī:

> Then mark with the blunt end of a probe [*mîl*] the site where you want to introduce the needle. This produces a depression [*djaouna*] and allows the point of the needle to enter without slipping. The cataract needle should be long enough to reach the pupil or should exceed it by the width of a barley corn, but not more.[301]

> If it is longer, attach something to it, preferably brass buttons [*rommânât min sofr*], which you can slide on or remove as you wish.[302]

> Now press the needle firmly enough until it perforates conjunctiva and cornea. The iris can be easily pushed backward so that it is not perforated by the instrument.[303]

---

specified as the visual target in both the Latin and Arabic. However, Hirschberg admitted that the parenthetical expression actually came from the Memorandum Book of Iba Isa, who does specify the nose as the target.

298 Personal communication, Oliver Kahl, 2020.

299 Meyerhof 1932.

300 Blodi et al. 1993, p. 294.

301 Hirschberg 1982, vol. 1, p. 348. Arabic transliterations from Meyerhof (1932). The term for probe (*mîl*) is from the Greek μήλη (Meyerhof 1932).

302 Feugère 1985. Based on the Arabic manuscripts of Antyllus, both Feugère (1985) and Meyerhof (1932) agreed that Antyllus recommended an adjustable metallic stop. Based on the Latin Continens, Hirschberg translated: "If the sharp end of the needle is longer than that distance then a thread should be wrapped around the needle so that it cannot be pushed too deeply into the eye. It is best if the instrument has a sheath so that the needles can be put in a container and taken out if needed." (Hirschberg 1985, vol. 2, p. 214) Hirschberg was perhaps being overly specific regarding the Latin as specifying threads, because the Continens actually mentions covering the needle with "something [*aliquid*]" (Rhazes 1529, p. 41). Hirschberg defended his interpretation of the Latin indumenta (*rumnanat* in Arabic) on the grounds that such sheaths have been found in the tombs of Gallo-Roman ophthalmologists (Hirschberg 1985, vol. 2, p. 214) After reviewing the Arabic manuscripts, Hirschberg translated: "If the needle is longer then cover part of it by a thread. The needle should be kept in a sheath [*indumenta, rumnanat*] of copper so that is can be withdrawn whenever you want to." (Hirschberg 1982, vol. 1, p. 348)

303 Hirschberg 1982, vol. 1, p. 349.

> The uvea [*'inabî*] is easily repelled, without being perforated, by the instrument, because it recedes because of its viscosity [*viscositatem, luzūğa*] and because the tip of the needle is not very sharp.[304]
>
> When the needle is now in the eye come closer with your mouth and then blow onto the eye of the patient so that the pupil remains regular [*recta*].[305]

Feugère agreed that the Latin *Continens* indicates blowing on the eye.[306] However, Meyerhof and Feugère read the Escorial manuscript to have Antyllus recommend placing the mouth on the eye and sucking until the pupil becomes normal (round).[307] Alternatively, the Arabic manuscripts used for the Indian edition of al-Rāzī recommend placing a piece of cotton on the eye.[308]

> Leave the instrument in its position and watch its tip. If it has not yet reached the cataract then push it a little forward. If it has been pushed beyond the cataract then retract it a little until it is on the same plane as the cataract.
>
> If you have achieved this then elevate the handle of the needle slowly, therefore the tip of the needle will be depressed. Do not cease this maneuver before the necessary result has been obtained and the cataract has been depressed into the depths of the eye.[309]
>
> If the cataract is difficult to remove and rises again then fragment the cataract toward the lateral or the nasal side whichever seems to be easier for the surgeon. This has to be repeated until the patient sees again. If this has been achieved withdraw the needle [*extrahatur instrumentum foris*].[310]
>
> Put for three days a compress of eggwhite with rose oil in the eye. The patient should always lie on his back. White ointment [*chiyâf*] should afterwards be put into the eye because he has pain in his eyes.[311]

---

304 Meyerhof 1932. In this case, the uveal tissue in question is the ciliary body or iris. In this case, the uveal tissue in question is the ciliary body or iris. According to Oliver Kahl (personal communication, 2021), the term translated as "viscosity" reads in the Arabic luzūğa; this word covers the semantic range of "viscidity, stickiness, glueyness" as well as "elasticity".

305 Hirschberg 1985, vol. 2, p. 215.

306 Feugère 1985.

307 Meyerhof 1932, Feugère 1985.

308 Feugère 1985.

309 Hirschberg 1982, vol. 1, p. 349.

310 Hirschberg 1985, vol. 2, pp. 214-216. The Latin passage in the Continens translated here as "withdraw the needle" was actually omitted from the Arabic (Meyerhof 1932).

311 Hirschberg 1985, vol. 2, pp. 214-216. Arabic transliteration from Meyerhof (1932).

Bandage the unoperated eye during the operation and also bandage it while the patient is lying on his back.[312]

He should remain in a dark room. He should be visited frequently to find out how he is feeling. The patient should avoid sneezing, talking and coughing. The bandage remains in place for three days except if there is a complication or necessity to remove it. If it should become necessary to reintroduce the instrument because the cataract has risen again we use the original opening; the opening does not close that quickly.[313]

Feugère 1985 identified another fragment from al-Rāzī in which Antyllus mentioned:

Sometimes you penetrate too far with the cataract needle; then blood pours out and remains in the eye's pupil, and an incurable condition arises.[314]

The cataract method of Antyllus was a seminal text underlying later descriptions by authors of medieval Arabic treatises of Ibn Isa, Ammar of Cairo, and Ibn Sina. For instance, both Antyllus and Ibn Sina mentioned releasing the cataract with an incision below the cornea, and both Antyllus and Ammar described aspiration of the cataract by suction.[315] We also see some overlap of the method of Antyllus with elements related to cataract surgery in the Ayurvedic and Chinese works.

## Placement of Metallic Rings to Widen the Shaft (250 CE)

The standard Greco-Roman metal couching needles prevented excessive entry by having a wider part of the shaft, which was a fixed part of the probe. In contrast, Antyllus in the Latin *Continens* indicated that the needle was covered with "something [*aliquid*]," without specifying the nature of the covering.[316] However, in surviving Arabic manuscripts of al-Rāzī, Antyllus specified that brass rings were placed.[317] Likewise, Salah al-Din wrote:

A collar ring should be attached to the needle separating the body of the needle from the point.[318]

---

312 Meyerhof 1932.

313 Hirschberg 1985, vol. 2, pp. 214-216. From the Latin Continens.

314 Feugère 1985.

315 A separate fragment of Antyllus from Rhazes Continens relating to cataract extraction and aspiration is discussed in later chapters of this book.

316 Rhazes 1529, p. 41.

317 Hirschberg 1982, vol. 1, p. 348. Feugère 1985. Based on the Arabic manuscripts of Antyllus, both Feugère (1985) and Meyerhof (1932) agreed that Antyllus recommended an adjustable metallic stop.

318 Blodi et al. 1993, p. 292.

Ammar of Cairo wrote: "A ring should be placed on the needle in order to separate the body of it from the needle."[319] Some Indian and later medieval Arabic works recommended wrapping the probe or a preliminary lancet in thread, rather than metallic rings.

## Turning the Eyes Medially (250 CE)

Having the patient turn the operative eye toward the medial canthus or the nose during cataract surgery, but to look laterally during pterygium surgery, is found in both Greco-Roman and Ayurvedic works. Given the difficulties in dating both Antyllus and the ophthalmic chapters of the *Suśrutasaṃhitā*, it is impossible to state whether this practice began closer to the Mediterranean or to India. Antyllus was the only Greek or Roman author to have the patient gaze medially during the cataract operation. In Antyllus' writing related to pterygium removal, there is no mention of the patient being asked to fixate on a visual target, but the brief surviving passage lacks detail.[320]

Ammar of Cairo had the cataract surgery patient look toward the nose but seemed to advise that the right hand be used in all cases.[321] Similarly, Ammar had the patient gaze laterally for pterygium surgery:

> When the assistant opens the eye, he should ask the patient to look towards the lateral canthus.[322]

Ibn Isa advised the surgeon to "Instruct the [cataract] patient to direct his gaze towards his nose."[323] Ibn Sina instructed the patient to look at both the medial canthus and the nose:

> Have the patient look towards the corner of his eye in front of the tearing side and look at his nose.[324]

When we consider surviving passages of Antyllus and derivative Arabic works as a group, we can identify having the patient look at both the medial canthus and the nose during cataract surgery and look laterally during pterygium surgery. These elements also feature prominently in the Ayurvedic works, as we describe in a subsequent chapter.

---

319  Blodi et al. 1993, p. 159.

320  Savage-Smith 1984.

321  Blodi et al. 1993, p. 152.

322  Hirschberg...Wafai 1993, p. 114.

323  Ibn Isa, Wood 1936, p. 184.

324  Ibn Sina, Sardo 2014 vol. 3, p. 273.

Having the cataract surgical patient gaze in a particular direction did not arrive in China until quite late. Moreover, instead of performing the paracentesis temporally, either a nasal or temporal approach was used, to allow the surgeon to easily use the right hand. The Yen K'e Ta Ch'uan *The Most Complete Eye Book*, written about 1628 CE in China, advised:

> The eye is opened by the operator with his thumb and index finger of the left hand... while operator's right hand holds the needle. If the right eye is operated upon, the patient must look toward the right; otherwise the bridge of the nose will interfere with the operation.[325]

# Cataracts Can Resemble Ice or Snow (250 CE)

Antyllus wrote that cataracts occurred from the cold and compared cataracts to snow [*niuis*].[326] Similarly, in the 6th century, Paulus Aegineta stated that some cataracts resembled a hailstone.

The Ayurvedic works do not compare cataracts to ice or snow. But this teaching might have traveled eastward along the Silk Road without leaving traces in the surviving Ayurvedic works. In China, the *Treatise of Bodhisattva Nagarjuna on Eye (Diseases)*, thought to be written by 907 CE (and published in 1445 CE), related the different types of cataract:

> There is rough, slippery or powdery one. The icy one when turned necessarily goes down, the slippery one does not cover (the pupil) firmly, and the rough screen could be dealt with a little late. The one that is powdery, when scraped, is very difficult to gather and remove.[327]

Another translation of this passage from the Chinese based on a manuscript in the Korean archives explicitly noted both icy and snowy types:

> ...cataract...can be divided morphologically into four types: 1) surface irregular or uneven type, 2) surface smooth type, 3) brittle ice type and 4) snow-white type.[328]

---

325 Pi 1929; Having the patient gaze at a particular target is not found in early Chinese works attributed to Nagarjuna (Deshpande, Fan 2012 Restoring the Dragon's Vision) or in Essential Subtleties on the Silver Sea.

326 Rhazes 1529, Book 2, capitulum 3, section QQ, car. 41, image 102. At our request, David Butterfield, PhD translated this paragraph.

327 Deshpande, Fan 2012, p. 109. Deshpande "Sino-Indian" 2000. Deshpande believes this text (*Longshu pusa yanlun*) was written by the end of the Tang era (618 to 907 CE).

328 *Longshu Pusa Yanlun*, Mishima 2004, pp. 88-89.

In Nagarjuna's Comprehensive Treatise, mentioned in 1111 CE and published in the 16th century, there was an icy "screen" (cataract) suitable for couching which involved pain, a red eye, and a white pupil:

> The icy screen is just like water refined and firm. It is like the yang within the yin.[329]

The same treatise also described a "powdered screen" (cataract), with a bluish-green and then white pupil. One was only able to see "the three lights." The disorder was treatable with "a golden needle."[330]

## Cataracts Can Be Too Hard for Couching (250 CE)

The Greco-Roman works (beginning with Antyllus) added that the cataract could be too hard to be reliably couched and that those of moderate consistence were ideal. According to al-Rāzī (Rhazes), Antyllus held that deformation of the cataract when the eye was rubbed, and the pupillary colors, were both relevant to assessment of cataract maturity.[331]

Paulus, Ibn Isa, and Ibn Sina followed Antyllus' teachings in this regard.[332] Ibn Isa wrote: "Furthermore the cataract should not be too dense or too watery."[333] Ibn Sina wrote of a cataract type: "so thick and hard that you cannot call it water. And this condition is not treatable."[334]

The unsuitability of the hard cataract for couching is found in the later Ayurvedic works of Vāgbhata. Among the types of cataract apparently unsuitable for couching (because they are not specified as caused by kapha), we find in the *Aṣṭāṅga Hṛdayam*:

> *Śarkarā* is that in which the vision (lens) appears as though smeared with milky sap of arka and is thick/hard.[335]

This idea is not apparent in the medieval Chinese works.

---

329 Deshpande, Fan 2012, p. 148. "Icy screen inner obstacle" also called *Bing yi nei zhang*.

330 Deshpande, Fan 2012, p. 152. "An internal obstacle due to the powdered screen," termed *San yi nei zhang*.

331 Rhazes 1529, Book 2, capitulum 3, section QQ, p. 41.

332 Paulus, Adams 1846, vol. 2, p. 279; ibn Isa, Wood 1936, p. 179.

333 Ibn Isa, Wood, 1936, p. 179.

334 Ibn Sina, Sardo 2014, p. 271.

335 Vagbhata, Murthy 2017 vol. III, Ch. 14, "Linganasa Pratsedha," p. 132.

# Marking with a Second Instrument (250 CE)

Starting with Antyllus, in the Greek works (and their Arabic successors), the use of the primary instrument is preceded by applying to the eye a different instrument (or the opposite end of the primary instrument). The purposes proposed for use of the other instrument grow progressively more aggressive: to mark the site of the puncture, to acclimatize the patient to the touch, and to make a small indentation in the conjunctiva where the primary rod will enter. Antyllus believed depressing with the blunt end of the probe [*mîl*] would produce a depression [*djaouna*] to prevent the needle from slipping.[336] Paul of Aegina marked the penetration spot with the knob of the *specillum* in the same way but did not explain the reason.[337] Ibn Isa believed, as Antyllus did, that marking would help the doctor place the needle and added that marking would help the patient's state of mind:

> Then measure with the end of the instrument at the margin of the cornea towards the external canthus and at the margin of the former, just where you will enter the tip, and there make an impression (mark or puncture)—a small pit. This slight cut will, first, try out the patient's endurance and gain his confidence; second, it will create a place for the point of the needle where it will have a firm hold, will not slip off the eyeball nor fail to enter or to be easily removed during the operation.[338]

In China, the *Treatise of Bodhisattva Nagarjuna on Eye (Diseases)*, thought to be written by 907 CE (and first published in 1445 CE), also emphasized that marking helped the patient remain calm:

> First with another blunt stick (needle) decide the point of piercing, then the eye gets used to it, since there is a fear of (patient getting) a fright and a sudden movement (by him) therefore it is necessary to determine the point of piercing beforehand.[339]

The 14th- or 15th-century Chinese treatise *Essential Subtleties on the Silver Sea* instructed: "Slowly determine with the blunt end of a bronze hairpin the position [where the needle] is to be inserted."[340] Marking of the spot for penetration is not explicitly mentioned in the Ayurvedic works of Suśruta or Vāgbhata.

---

336  Hirschberg 1982, vol. 1, p. 348. Arabic transliterations from Meyerhof (1932). The term for probe (*mîl*) is from the Greek μήλη (Meyerhof 1932).

337  Paulus, Adams 1846, p. 280.

338  Ibn Isa, Wood 1936, p. 184.

339  Deshpande, Fan 2012, p. 110. Deshpande "Sino-Indian" 2000. Deshpande believes this text (*Longshu pusa yanlun*) was written by the end of the Tang era (618 to 907 CE).

340  Kovacs, Unschuld 1998, p. 404. *Yin-hai jing-wei.*

## Vision Testing (250 CE)

Antyllus recommended pushing the cataract down until the patient could see.[341] However, Paulus Aegineta specifically advised against early vision testing because the exertion could cause the cataract to reascend.[342] Ibn Isa believed that the patch over the sound eye was useful so that "in testing recovered vision immediately after the operation one can be certain the patient is not looking with his sound eye."[343] Albucasis in the 10th century noted: "If the humour comes down at once, the patient will at once see whatever his vision is opened upon while the needle is still in his eye."[344]

The Ayurvedic works also recommended vision testing during and immediately after surgery. The Chinese text *Treatise of Bodhisattva Nagarjuna on Eye (Diseases)* noted that just after needle removal but before bandage placement: "When the eye is opened after a long time, it is as if seeing things in a bright clear light."[345] Similarly, *Essential Subtleties on the Silver Sea* noted:

> When the needling is completed, the [patient] may recline. Remove the paper, take something into your hand and let the patient look at it. The patient will [be able to] see it. Do not let the patient look at bystanders for too long.[346]

Testing the vision immediately after couching was performed in Tibet in the 20th century (Figs. 17, 18).[347]

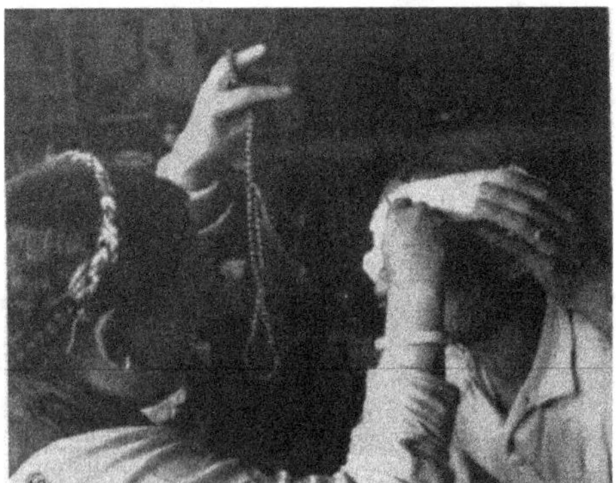

**Fig. 17.** A Tibetan oculist tests vision with her necklace just after couching a cataract in 1955.

---


341 Feugère 1985.

342 Paulus, Adams 1846, vol. 2, p. 280.

343 Ibn Isa, Wood 1936, p. 184.

344 Albucasis et al. 1973, p. 252.

345 *Longshu pusa yanlun.* Deshpande, Fan "Restoring the Dragon's Vision" 2012, p. 111.

346 Kovacs, Unschuld 1998, p. 404.

347 Rambo 1955.

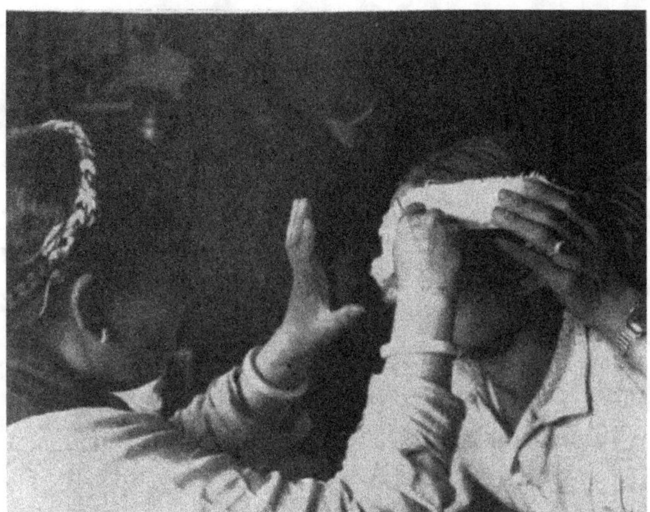

**Fig. 18.** A Tibetan oculist tests vision with her fingers just after couching a cataract in 1955.

## Placing Cotton and Blowing on the Eye (250 CE)

In the *Book of Tobit*, Tobias healed his father's eyes by blowing on them while applying fish gall. Blowing on the eye was practiced by indigenous New World healers and is probably many thousands of years old.[348]

The materials placed on the eye during treatment varied by location, with Celsus in Europe placing wool (*lana*), near Eastern or Indian doctors placing cotton, and Chinese doctors placing "moist paper."[349] Linen was also used in some ophthalmic healing by Celsus (*linum, linamentum*) and Aëtius of Amida.

The works of Antyllus, and derivative Arabic works, recommend placing cotton on the eye and blowing in the eye, often in conjunction. Ibn Isa of medieval Baghdad put cotton on the eye and then blew on the cotton not once, but twice. The first time was to preoperatively assess the maturity of the cataract by:

> ...laying a cotton-wool pad over the eye to be observed and blowing on it forcibly with one's own hot breath. Then examine the eye uncovered; if the cataract appears to move and seems clear, it is an indication for operation.[350]

Ibn Isa repeated the practice while the needle was in the eye:

348  Leffler et al. 2017.
349  Kovacs, Unschuld 1998, Essential Subtleties on the Silver Sea, p. 404.
350  Ibn Isa, Wood 1936, p. 180.

> The eye that is being operated on should at this stage be covered with a layer of fresh cotton wool on which you should audibly blow warm breaths of air and make sounds like drinking, as if to relieve the unrest of the eye.[351]

Zayn al-Din Sayyed Isma'il ibn Husayn Gorgani (c. 1040-1136) was from Gorgon, but later moved to Merv, in today's Kazakhstan. Gorgani (or Jurjani) in 1110 wrote a medical treatise called *Zakhireye Khwarazmshahi* for Qutb ad-Din Muhammad, the first Shah of Khwarezm. Jurjani rendered this passage (book 6, chapter 2):

> Place a piece of clean wool over the eye and blow gently upon it. Or place your mouth near to the eye and inhale as though taking a drink.[352]

Ibn Sina (Avicenna) repeated Ibn Isa's test of maturity by placing cotton on the eye and blowing on it:

> Put some cotton on the eye and blow it fast and then take the cotton away and check the eye immediately and without delay. See if the water has moved, and if it has moved, that is a sign that you can take it out easily.[353]

Two 12th century authors in Italy, Master Zachary, who trained in Constantinople, and David Armenicus, who claimed to have lived in Baghdad and drawn on Indian sources, both recommended that the ophthalmologist chew fennel, cumin or other substances, and then blow on the eye during cataract surgery. Zachary wrote "... et tu accipias feniculum vel semen ejus, et sal, et ciminum, et mastica inter dentes, et eis in ore existentibus, banela fortiter contra oculum patientis satis quantum tibi visum fuerit." David wrote "Quando vero volueris percutere cataractam, primo magister accipiat semen feniculi, et ponat in ore, et masticet ipsum semen, et de flatu suo debeat emanare in oculo infirmantis."[354] The Latin *Continens* of Rhazes provides Antyllus' method, in which the operator blows on the eye with the needle in place.[355] Others agree that the Latin *Continens* indicates blowing on the eye.[356] However, Meyerhof and Feugère read the Escorial Arabic manuscript to have Antyllus recommend placing the mouth on the eye and sucking until the pupil becomes normal (round).[357] Alternatively, the Arabic manuscripts used for the Indian edition of al-Rāzī recommend placing a piece of cotton on the eye.[358] These variant readings of Antyllus (blowing, sucking, placing cotton) must be interpreted in light of the works of Ibn Isa and Avicenna, in which placing cotton on the eye and blowing are performed in conjunction. With the close connection between these works, it seems

---

351 Ibn Isa, Wood 1936, p. 185.

352 Elgood 1970, pp. 57, 64-66.

353 Ibn Sina, Sardo 2014, vol. 3, p. 271.

354 Pansier 1903-8, pp. 39

355 Hirschberg, Blodi 1985, vol. 2, p. 215.

356 Feugère 1985.

357 Meyerhof 1932; Feugère 1985.

358 Feugère 1985.

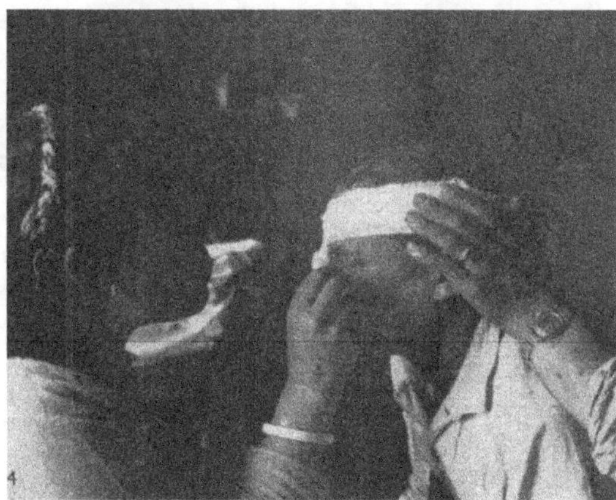

**Fig. 19.** A Tibetan oculist blows on the operative eye while the couching needle is still embedded in the eye in 1955.

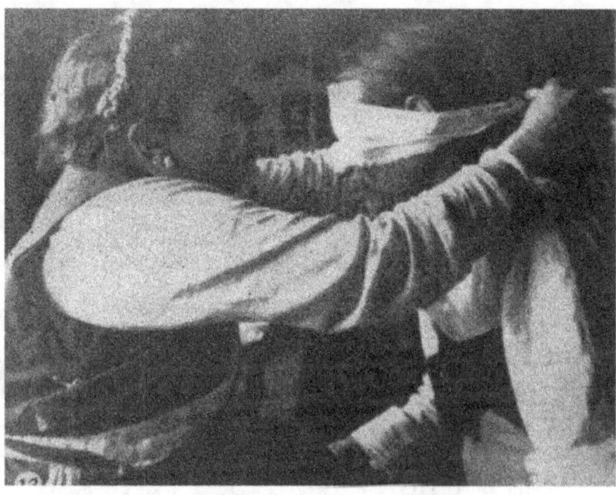

**Fig. 20.** A cataract patient from Tibet has his operative eye bandaged with sheep's wool at the end of the case. Wool, as opposed to cotton, was the personal preference of the oculist.

likely that Antyllus did recommend placing cotton on the eye and blowing on the eye. (Perhaps, the sucking recommended by Antyllus corresponds with Ibn Isa's "make sounds like drinking.")

The use of cotton has a long history by the inhabitants along the greater Indus Valley region.[359] In the Ayurvedic works, blowing on the eye and placing cotton on it were both performed during cataract surgery, but not simultaneously. Vāgbhata I blew on the eye preoperatively: "...blow warm air on the eye."[360] In India, "fomenting" the eye with heat was held to be beneficial from antiquity up to the modern period. Cotton was applied after the procedure, similar to how we place a patch today: "...a swab of cotton soaked in comfortable warm ghee is placed on the eye and the

---

359 Moulherat 2002.

360 Vāgbhata, Murthy 2000, vol. 3, p. 150. *Aṣṭāṅgasaṃgraha* 6.17.7.

bandage applied…"[361] As described by Breton,[362] simultaneous fomentation of the eye and placement of cotton near the eye, both while the probe was still embedded, survived in India into the 19th century. Blowing while the couching instrument was in the eye was still practiced in Tibet in the 20th century (Figs. 19 and 20).[363]

Greek sources (as Indian) would deliver medicines by blowing them.[364] But to treat a disorder just by blowing on the eye was more consistent with traditional Indian medicine. Suśruta noted: "…in case of minute foreign bodies in sense organs, it should be cleaned with washing and blowing and with hairs (brush), cloth and hands…"[365] For a traumatized eye, Suśruta recommended: "The injured eye becomes painless on fomenting it slightly with mouth-vapour."[366]

## Publius Flavius Vegetius Renatus (late 4th century)

In his veterinary work, primarily related to horses, Vegetius describes medical treatment of ocular suffusions with opobalsamum. Suitable suffusions (cataracts) could be couched:

Of couching the Eye. But if the strength of a distemper has brought a blindness or a suffusion into the eye, observe carefully what colour the membrane [*membrana*] is…If it be of the colour of gold [*auroso*], you may know it to be incurable; if it be too white [*candida*], you shall also know that you cannot cure it. But if it be thick, of an olive [*oleagino*] colour, like mucus [*muco*], it is cured by couching [*paracenthesim*], after it is ripened [*maturata*], just after the same manner as that of men. Therefore the day before, you shall keep the horse from food, but especially restrain him from drinking; you shall throw him down in a soft place, and place his head and his neck commodiously; you shall open his eye so wide that he may not be able to shut it, then you shall put in the couching instrument by the very front or fore-part between the coats of the eye, so as not to touch the pupil of the eye, or hurt any thing in the inside of it, but with the head of the couching instrument [*paracenterium*] depress the white [*album*] itself from the upper part, where the suffusion [*hypochysis*] is placed, nicely downwards to the lower eyelid; and if it be couched or put down, you must not take out the couching instrument before you have for a very long while vaporated [*vaporaveris*] the closed eye with a warm spunge, for it uses to start back again; and if it shall so happen, repress it, till it be so fixed and put in such order, that it may not be able to start back again. When therefore you shall perceive that the clearness and brightness of the pupil of the eye receives no manner of obstacle from the suffusion [*hypochysis*], you shall then take out the iron [*ferrum*] instrument,

---

361 Vāgbhata, Murthy 2000, vol. 3, p. 151. *Aṣṭāṅgasaṃgraha* 6.17.10.

362 Breton 1826.

363 Rambo 1955.

364 Hirschberg, Blodi 1982, vol. 1, pp. 191,210.

365 Susruta, Sharma 2018, vol. 1, p. 275; Sushruta, Bhishagratna 1907, vol. 1, p. 257.

366 Suśruta, Sharma 2014, vol. 3, p. 229. (SS 6.19.5)

and you shall find that the animal does actually see [*videre*]. You shall dress it after this manner; you shall make a conglutinating composition with the oil of roses, and the white of an egg, soak wool in it, and put it upon the eye after you have couched it, and over all bind it up with a bandage.[367]

The incurability of the golden pupil echoes the text of Celsus.

# A humor Descending from the Brain into the Eyes (Late 4th Century)

Several centuries into the Common Era, we find the idea that some sort of fluid descending from the brain into the eyes produces the lesion treated by couching. As we saw in the section on phlegm, the Hippocratic work *Diseases 2* referred to phlegm, which, in context, seemed to be descending from the brain to the eyes to blur vision. However, as this section of the work is considered to post-date the Hippocratic era, the passage is difficult to date.

Elsewhere, the Hippocratic text *Places in Man* described a fluid descending from the brain to the eye, but this seemed to be a physiologic occurrence:

...narrow vessels lead to the pupil from the brain...These vessels nourish the pupil with purest moisture the brain, and it is in this moisture that he image appears in the eyes. The same vessels also extinguish the pupils if they dry out...The pupil is nourished by moisture from the brain; if it takes up anything from the vessels, it is disturbed by this afflux, and the image does not appear normally in it...[368]

Galen described a functional *pneuma* that descended from the brain into the eyes, but this was a physiologic carrier of information, and its obstruction was observed within eyes with cataracts. Galen also wrote in *On the Causes of Symptoms* that a cataract was due to a thickened aqueous humor, but he did not say it resulted from a descent of fluid into the eye.[369]

But at least by the late 4th century, authors describe a pathologic humor that descends from the brain into the eyes to produce cataracts. Vegetius wrote that with respect to suffusions: "...a *Hypocoriasis* proceeds from a Humour of the Head that descends into it..."[370] About 500 CE, the Bava Kamma of the Babylonian Talmud

---

367 Book 2, chap. 17. Vegetius 1748, pp. 150-152. Latin: Vegetius 1574, p. 71; and Paulus, Adams 1846, vol. 2, p. 283.

368 Hippocrates, Potter, 1995, vol. VIII, Places in Man, LCL 482, pp. 22-25.

369 Galen, Johnston, On Diseases and Symptoms, 2006, p. 210. Pupillary reflexes are discussed in a subsequent chapter.

370 Vegetius 1748, p. 149.

stipulated that brain injuries caused blindness by causing fluid to flow from the brain to cover the eye.[371]

Hunain in the 10th century wrote of visual symptoms (not due to cataracts), which resulted from fumes coming from the brain:

> The phantasms originating in the brain are caused by the disease the Greek name of which is *phrenitis*...when the hot dry chyme in the brain is burnt by the heat of fevers, there rises from it a fume like that of oil burnt in the fire. When this fume penetrates the eye by the arteries leading to it from the brain, it produces in it the various kinds of phantasms.[372]

Ibn Isa in 11th-century Baghdad falsely attributed this teaching to Galen:

> Galen in the fourth book on Causes and Symptoms teaches that when the albuminous humor becomes thick (inspissated) it is due to a descent of fluid into the eye. A 'descent of water' is the Arabic technical term for 'formation of cataract'.[373]

Ammar of 11th-century Cairo believed that cataracts were due to something descending from the brain, which was closer to a fluid than to a vapor:

> For the origin of the cataract in the eye is a fine effusion which accumulates (condenses) out of a very damp mist under the involvement of the brain, which reaches a state of humid dyscrasia. It thus slowly thickens in the eye...That is why the descending of the cataract into the eye and blurring of vision in the affected eye only takes a month or two in some cases...[374]

In the Chinese literature, the humor that flowed down from the brain to cause cataracts has sometimes been translated as "fat." In the text *Wai Tai Mi Yaofang*, Wang Tao (d. 755 CE) cited "The Discussion of Eyes" in the Indian classic by Xie Daoren, who described a disease called *nao liu qing mang* ("the flow of brain into the eyes causes blindness").[375] In the early 9th-century *Treatise of Bodhisattva Nagarjuna on Eye (Diseases)*, the discussion of cataract couching explained:

> The cataract could be either old (mature) or tender (immature). According to (the kind of) damage, *qi* and natural character, a person contracts excessive heat and the brain (fat) flows down forming an obstruction then it is easy to reduce.[376]

---

371 Gordon 1933. This is mentioned in the Babylonian Talmud in the Bava Kamma 98a (450 CE-550 CE).

372 Hunain, Meyerhof 1928, p. 71.

373 Ibn Isa, Wood 1936, p. 179.

374 Blodi et al. 1993, pp. 147-148.

375 Ka Wai Fan 2005.

376 Deshpande, Fan 2012, pp. 108-109.

78

In the Ayurvedic literature, cataracts are clearly due to humors, but it is not specifically stated that these pathologic humors arise from the stomach, or are descending from the brain into the eye.

# On the Etymology of the Term Cataract (5th Century)

In Latin, the term *cataracta* came to replace *suffusio* to represent an intraocular opacity obscuring vision. Fischer has identified multiple early Latin uses of the term *cataracta* in an ophthalmic sense. Perhaps the earliest identified use of the term is the section title (*De cataractis*) of a copy of Celsus' *De Medicina,* which might date from the early 5th century.[377] The term also appears in the 6th-century Latin texts of Gregory of Tours, France, and in *Sapientia Artis Medicinae.* A Latin translation of Oribasius, which also might date from the 6th-century, translated ὑπόχυσιν [*hypochysin*] as "*ypocisin, id est cataractas*". In addition, ὑποχύσεις [*hypochyseis*] was rendered "*catharactas*". A Latin commentary on the Hippocratic aphorism 6:56, in a 10th-century manuscript believed to record commentary originally from the 8th or 9th century in France, explained that "*cataracta*" was one type of blindness.[378] The codex London Arundel 166 is a 9th-century manuscript from France or Germany, the first part of which contains text attributed to Pliny and Celsus. The second half, which contains prescriptions by Scribonius Largus and Marcellus Empiricus, contains a recipe for a collyrium including opobalsamum for "*cataractas*", which suddenly cause vision loss.[379] Another 9th-century manuscript, the cod. Vat. Reg. lat. 1143, contains a medical treatment for "*cataraptas*", which gradually cause vision loss.[380]

In summary, the term *cataracta* was used in medieval Latin as an equivalent for the Greek *hypochyma*, from the 5th to 9th centuries, though all known surgical discussions of *cataracta* date from the 5th and 6th centuries. When Constantine the African used the term *cataracta* to translate the Arabic term "water" for cataract in 11th-century Salerno, he was using a term with a long tradition in Latin Europe.

The term *cataract* was used in ancient Latin and Greek to represent something that moved down—either a waterfall, a portcullis, water sluice, floodgate, drawbridge, or a waterbird that descended quickly. Given Gregory of Tours' description of ophthalmic cataracts as both descending, and being able to be opened, one possible interpretation is that he thought of the disorder as a portcullis. In classical Latin, "*Cataracta clausa erat*" means "The portcullis had been closed."[381] An interpretation

---

377 Fischer 2000, p. 127. Unfortunately, Fischer's important work has been almost undiscovered in the English literature.

378 Fischer 2000, p. 127.

379 Fischer 2000, p. 127. On folio 14R of Lond. Arundel 166. The same material is also on the manuscript Echternacher Handschrift Par. Lat. 11219. Lond. Arundel 166 information from www.bl.uk.

380 Fischer 2000, p. 127. Folio 175 r-v of the codex.

381 Livy, Moore 1943, pp. 324-325.

as a waterfall would require a bit of figurative imagination, as we do not usually speak of opening waterfalls.

Still, perhaps some imagination is in order. The bulk of the texts, from the 5th-century edition of Celsus, straight through to Constantine in the 11th century, equated *cataracta* with the Greek *hypochyma*, and ultimately with the corresponding Arabic term "water." *Hypochyma* is related to a fluid that had settled in the eye, obscuring vision. We might presume that ophthalmic use of the term arose in Late Latin, given its apparent absence in ancient and medieval Greek texts.

Later in the Middle Ages, authors guessed at a variety of etymologies of the term *cataract*. Gilbert thought it might be derived from the word characters.[382] Of course, it was easy to guess that the cataract might relate to a waterfall, given its nonophthalmic uses of the term in antiquity, its often-white appearance in the eye, like a waterfall, and the conjunction with the Arabic understanding of a cataract as water in the eye. Velasco de Tharanta (1382-1417) wrote in the *Philonium*: "... so is a cataract in the eye from the coldness of the brain...This is why the ancients named it in analogy with falling water."[383]

## Gregory of Tours (6th century)

Gregory of Tours (538-594) used the term *cataract* to describe eye ailments several times. The cataract descended upon the eye:

> Here I will expound only what has happened to the negligent, who after the virtue of heaven have sought out earthly medicaments, because his virtue is demonstrated not only in the methods of his cures but also in his punishing the stupid. Leonastis, Archdeacon of Bourges, lost the sight of his eyes when cataracts descended [*decedentibus cataractis*] upon him. And when he could not receive any vision at all as he went around many doctors, he went to the basilica of St Martin; there he remained for two or three months, fasted continually, and prayed for the recovery of his sight. And indeed when the festival arrived, his eyes were made clear and he began to see; and when he had returned home, he summoned a Jew and put cupping glasses on his shoulders, by whose help he could increase the sight in his eyes. And when his blood also fell, he was again returned to a revived state of blindness.[384]

The ophthalmic cataract was also mentioned in conjunction with surgery to pierce the eyes, even if in the Christian view a miracle was superior to surgery. Gregory of Tours wrote:

---

382  Demaitre 2013, p. 165.

383  Demaitre 2013, pp. 165-166. From: *Practica que alias Philonium dicitur*.

384  Translation by David Butterfield, PhD, personal communication, 2014. In Latin: Gregory of Tours 1886, Book 5, Col. 210. p. 152.

> The deacon Theudomer suffered from a swelling on his head; when cataracts developed, the openings to his eyes were painfully blocked for four years.[385]

But then Theudomer knelt all night and shed tears on the ground.

> When daylight came, the cataracts on his eyes were opened [*reseratis cataractis luminum*], and he deserved to see the daylight. What [cure] such as this one have doctors ever accomplished with their implements? Their efforts produce more pain than healing; and after stretching and piercing an eye with their needles [*spiculis oculo*] they fashion the torments of death before they open the eye. If caution is lacking in this operation, the doctor is providing eternal blindness for the wretched patient.[386]

Gregory used the term *cataractis* with respect to the eyes at least 3 times and always in the phrases *decedentibus/decidentibus cataractis* or *reseratis cataractis*.[387]

## Paul of Aegina (6th century)

In the 6th century, Paul of Aegina compiled Greek cataract couching methods, citing Galen by name, and also probably borrowing from Antyllus:

> The cataract is a collection of inert fluids upon the cornea at the pupil, obstructing vision or preventing distinct vision. It arises most commonly from a congelation and weakness of the visual spirit, and on that account the disease rather attacks old persons, and those who are debilitated by protracted illness. It is occasioned also by violent vomiting, a blow, and many other causes. Those kinds of cataract which are not but commencing, as not being proper objects of surgery, have been treated of in the Third Book. We shall now give the characters of those which are fairly formed and have acquired consistence. All those, therefore, who have cataract see the light more or less, and by this we distinguish cataract from amaurosis and glaucoma; for persons affected with these complaints do not see the light at all. Wherefore, again, Galen well instructs us as to the consistence and difference of cataracts and which kinds ought to be operated upon. Having shut the eye affected with the cataract, and with the large finger pressing the eyelid to the eye, and moving it with pressure to this side and that, then opening the eyelids and observing the cataract in the eye; if it has not yet acquired consistence, a certain flow takes place from the pressure of the finger, and at first it appears broader, but straightway resumes its former figure and magnitude. But in those which have acquired consistence no change takes place as to breadth or figure from the pressure. But since this appearance is common to those which are of moderate consistence, and those which are over-compacted, we distinguish these cases from one another by their colour. For those which are

---

385  Wallis 2010, p. 57.
386  Wallis 2010, p. 57. Latin in McVaugh 2001.
387  McVaugh 2001.

of an iron, coerulean [κυανόχροα, *kuanochroa*], or leaden colour, are of moderate consistence, and fit for couching; but those which resemble gypsum and hailstones are over-compacted. After ascertaining these circumstances, as directed by Galen, having placed the patient opposite the light, but not in the sun, we bind up carefully the sound eye, and having separated the lids of the other, at the distance from the part called the iris towards the small [lateral] canthus, of about the size of the knob of the specillum, we then with the point of the perforator mark the place about to be perforated; if it it is the left eye we operate with the right hand, or if the right eye with the left; and turning round the point of the perforator, which is bent at its extremity, we push it strongly through the part which was marked out, until we come to an empty place [κενεμβατήσεως, *kenembateseos*]. The depth of the perforation should be as great as the distance of the pupil from the iris. Wherefore, raising the perforator to the apex of the cataract, (for the copper of it is seen through the transparency of the cornea,) we push down the cataract to the parts below, and if it is immediately carried downwards, we rest for a little, but if it reascends we press it back again. After the depression of the cataract we turn round the perforator and extract it gently. After this, bathing with water and injecting into the eye a little Cappadocian salts, we apply externally some wool soaked in the white of an egg with rose-oil, and bind it up, and at the same time bind up the sound eye, that it may not move. Then lodging the patient in an apartment below ground, we order him to remain in a state of perfect rest, and upon a spare diet; and the bandages are to be kept on, if nothing prevent, until the seventh day, after which we loose them, and make trial of the sight by presenting him with some object: but this we disapprove of during the operation and immediately after it, lest by the intense exertion the cataract reascend. If the inflammation become urgent we loose the dressing before the seventh day, and must direct our attention to it.[388]

## *Sapientia Artis Medicinae* (6th century)

The medieval text *Sapientia Artis Medicinae* (Wisdom of the Art of Medicine) is thought to date from the 6th century, though the earliest manuscripts are from the 10th or 11th century. Most of the manuscripts just have portions of the text, rather than the entire composite text as presented in 1928. The section on cataracts has a paragraph that uses the Greek term for cataracts (*hypochymata*), followed by a method using the term observed in Latin-speaking areas (*cataractas*). Thus, the composite text may have drawn on the work of sources that were originally separate. This text is one of the few early medieval Latin texts to use the term *cataracta* to describe cataracts. The work recommends couching in the warmer seasons.

The human eye has seven tunics and there are seven cataracts [hypochymata]. All their names are written here: *platorides*, silver [*argyriides*], *graides*, *molydites*, *amaurosis*, *placodes*, *serotaxis*. You couch [*paracintidas*] *platorides* in the sixth year, silver [*argyriides*] in the eighth year and in the third year, if the person is old.

---

388  Paulus, Adams 1846, vol. 2, pp. 279-280. Greek from: Paulus, Heiberg, CMG, 1924, pp. 59-61.

You couch *graides* in the fourth year, and *placodes* in the second year. And if you find *molybdites*, *amaurosin*, and *serotaxis*, these are incurable.

Cure cataracts [*cataractas*] in the month of May [*maio*] and all summer and autumn. But when winter comes, leave off curing the eye. Cure cataracts [*cataractam*] like this: first you give to the stomach a cathartic of the sacred and bitter medicine [*hierapigra*]. After the third day you bleed the patient from the cephalic vein. After the fourth day, you tie his hands to his right knee. You couch [*paracintidas*] his left eye with your right hand. Couch him carefully, to avoid touching the sense of sight and taking out the eye. Another person should hold his head firmly so that it does not move, to avoid danger. Administer clean salty brine to the eyes and again place egg yolk over the eyes with soft wool [*lana mollissima*]. Let him lie in a secluded place [*loco secreto*] for nine days, so that he does not hear any noise. Twice daily, you will treat his stomach with a clyster. For his food, let him have new eggs and also barley-water. Refrain from wine and let him drink hot water for nine days, and on the tenth, let him have a bath and he will be better.[389]

# Cataracts Resembling Silver Can be Couched (6th century)

Earlier, we noted that, in the precouching era, Hippocrates observed that silvery pupils do not function. Moreover, in *Sapientia Artis Medicinae* of the 6th century, the silver (*argyriides*) cataract would be couched in the eighth year. The comparison of cataracts to silver is not found in the Ayurvedic literature, but does appear in the 12th-century Nagarjuna's Comprehensive Treatise from China:

Internal obstacle due to floating screen...It is like a silver needle in color...This eye should be pierced and (the obstacle) removed by turning with a golden needle.[390]

The 15th-century Chinese treatise *Essential Subtleties on the Silver Sea* was said by an editor in 1781 to derive its name because Daoist writings compare the eye to a silver sea.[391]

---

389 English translation adapted from Wallis 2010, pp. 17-20. Latin from Wlachsky 1928. An analysis of the various cataract colors mentioned has been published (Leffler, Klebanov et al. 2020, p. 80).

390 Deshpande, Fan 2012, pp. 153-154. Treatise *Longmu zong lun*. Disorder name *Fu yi nei zhang*.

391 Kovacs, Unschuld 1998, pp. 122-124. Treatise *Yin-hai jing-wei*.

# Collapse of Ophthalmology in the Medieval West (7th to 11th centuries)

Couching was described in ancient Greece and Rome. However, mentions of cataract surgery in medieval Western Europe are few and far between. Did cataract surgery spread northward, possibly as far as Roman Britain, and then recede or even disappear with the empire's collapse?

There seems to be a medieval gap in the descriptions of cataract couching in Europe. The shortest gap, of just two centuries, from the 9th to 11th centuries, occurs in the Byzantine literature. This short gap might suggest continuity of surgical practice in the Byzantine world.

On the other hand, consider the Iberian Peninsula. The Visigothic kingdom with its capitol at Toledo issued law codes in 654 and 681, which established:

> If a physician lifts from the eyes the *hypochyma* or removes it from the eyes and re-establishes the health of the patient then five solidi should be paid as his fee.[392]

The next mention of ophthalmic surgery in the area comes three centuries later. In 941, the Andalusian brothers Ahmad and 'Umar felt it necessary to travel to Baghdad to study the works of Galen and to train in the treatment of eye diseases, only returning in 962.[393] The contemporaneous writings of the Andalusian author al-Zahrawi (936-1013), known later as Albucasis, of Córdoba, suggest a personal familiarity with cataract couching.[394]

The Iberian Peninsula was reconquered by the Christians in the 15th century, until the last Arabic kingdom at Granada fell in 1492. During this century, much of the ophthalmic care was provided by Jewish oculists. For instance, in 1434 in Portugal, Master Nacim, a Jewish master in the art of the eyes *"mestre na arte dos olhos"* demonstrated his cures (*"curas"*) in Lisbon, where he resided,[395] and received a "Letter of Privilege," which entitled him to examine anyone else in the country who desired to practice this art.[396] In 1464, Mestre Daniel Colobro, a Jewish resident of Lisbon, declared that he was a servant and helper of Master Nacim.[397] In 1412, "maestre Manuel" who called himself *"físico de los ojos"* in Murcia complained to the town council that he had converted from Judaism to Catholicism to save his

---

392 Hirschberg, Blodi 1985, Vol. 2, p. 245. The code of 654 was the lawbook of Reccesvind (Recceswinth, Reccessvind) entitled "Antigua" or "Lex Visigothorum Reccesvindiana". The law was repeated in the Lex Visigothorum Erwigiana of 681.

393 Ibn Abī 'Uṣaybïa, Kopf 2017, p. 490.

394 Albucasis et al. 1973.

395 Carvalho 1939.

396 Collins 2020.

397 Carvalho 1939.

soul, but he earned less with the Christians. The council agreed to pay Manuel a salary.[398] In 1468, the Jewish rabbi and oculist of Lleida (Lerida), Cresques Abiabar successfully performed cataract couching on King Juan II of Aragón on September 11 and October 12, 1468.[399] In the 1470s, Leal, a Jewish woman of Seville, practiced ophthalmology. Her husband was a silversmith. She was called *"maestra* of healing eyes" and *"doña"*. Contracts from 1474 to 1478 for her healing with medications for unmarried daughters of a Muslim bricklayer, a sailor, and a farmer have survived. After 1478, when the Inquisition began in Seville, Leal is not heard from again.[400] When the Jews were expelled from Spain in 1492, there may have been some decline in Spanish ophthalmology. One cannot be absolutist about this assessment, because there was a law referencing *"oculistas"* in Simancas in 1510-1513,[401] and a law decreed by King Felipe II in 1588 licensing surgeons who treated *"cataratas"*.[402] Still, we do not have concrete examples of ophthalmologists in Spain again until 1590, when the Valencia authorities hired Pedro del Río, a "foreigner" surgeon, who cured cataracts, other eye diseases, and genitourinary disorders. He received a fixed salary in exchange for free treatment of the poor.[403]

The longest gap in known evidence of cataract surgery, of five centuries, appears elsewhere in the lands of the Western Roman Empire after its fall. Cataract couching is written about in the 6th-century text *Sapientia Artis Medicinae*. Next, we see cataract couching written about by the translator Constantine the African in 11th-century Salerno. Even these translations do not prove the actual presence of the procedure. A later ophthalmic author, Master Zacharias, was not able to study ophthalmology in Salerno or learn from Latin texts. Therefore, he trained in Constantinople under Theophilus, physician to the Emperor Manuel I Komnenos (reign 1143-1180), and wrote a text clearly influenced by Arabic teachings.[404]

As we covered elsewhere, surgical instruments consistent with couching needles were found in Roman Britain. If cataract surgery persisted after the Roman period in Britain, the practice was probably negatively impacted by the Council of Tours of 1163, which forbid the clergy from practicing medicine, and also by the expulsion of the Jews from Britain in 1290. We do not again find evidence of cataract surgery on the British Isles until the 1560s.[405]

---

398 Torres Fontes 1973, p. 240.

399 The doctor was also known as Ibn Abiatar Crescas, don Abiatar Aben-Crexcas. Cardoner i Planas 1973, pp. 174-176; Koren 1973, p. 4; Ruben Maslaton 2014; Balaguer 1862 p. 608; Hirschberg, Blodi 1985, vol. 2, p. 258.

400 Marquez de Aracena 2012.

401 Gonzalez Arce 2011.

402 Cobo 2004.

403 Terrada 2002.

404 Lascaratos 1998, p. 391. Hirschberg, Blodi 1985, vol. 2, pp. 254, 257. Name given as Magister Zacharias, Master Zacharias, Magistri Zacharie. Zacharias book, apparently published the year after Hirschberg wrote, was: Tractatus de passionibus oculorum: qui vocatur sisilacera: id est, secreta secretorum. Compilatus circa annos 1143-1180.

405 Leffler et al. 2021.

One historian has written that "...cataract was a condition ignored by the earliest surgical writers of the High Middle Ages [1000-1300 CE], and there is no good evidence that it was diagnosed and treated before the thirteenth century."[406] Perhaps, this historian is correct to imply that the procedure was not performed, but we must also consider the possibility that couching persisted at a low level without new observations being recorded. Clerics might have ascribed cures to miracles, rather than secular procedures, as proposed previously.[407] The ancient descriptions might have been dutifully copied without modification because the specifics of the procedures had not changed. This question is deserving of further scholarship.

A similar collapse might have taken place in Mesopotamia after 1258 when Baghdad was sacked by the Mongol leader Hulagu Khan. Libraries were destroyed. Our search for oculists turned up one who probably overlapped with the sack of Baghdad: Saʻd (ʻIzz al-Dawla) b. Manṣūr b. Kammūna (d. 1284) of Baghdad was a Jewish philosopher and physician who wrote a book about eye diseases quoted by Íadaqa al-Shādhilī of Cairo (14th century). ʻIzz al-Dawla was threatened with execution for criticizing Islam but was saved by the governor of Baghdad. He converted to Islam in 1280.[408] Then we do not hear of another oculist in Mesopotamia for over 400 years. Between 1732 and 1735, Regina Salomea Pilsztynowa, a woman oculist from Poland, explained she had learned from her oculist husband and "I gained some other useful information from another oculist, a Turk from Babylon" while in Istanbul.[409]

Constantinople fell to the Ottoman Empire in 1453. The Italian anatomist Alessandro Benedetti (c. 1450-1512) spent 16 years practicing in Morea in southern Greece and in Crete. He found that in Greece, there were few oculists and physicians because the Turks had destroyed the Greek educational system.[410]

It is easy to understand how complex projects such as the Roman aqueducts could not be built without large-scale social organization and would fall into disrepair during the Middle Ages. How cataract surgery, a procedure that can be performed with a thorn and that was often transmitted from fathers to sons, could disappear from a society is harder to understand. Nonetheless, it seems that when educational systems are destroyed, or particular social groups are targeted, it is possible for technical skills to disappear.

---

406 McVaugh 2001.

407 Lascaratos 1992, p. 145.

408 Lev 2021, p. 99.

409 Konczacki 2002; Pilsztynowa 2021, p. 75.

410 Lind 1975, p. 70.

# Ophthalmology in Constantinople
# (7th to 15th centuries)

Some ophthalmic cures in early medieval China were performed by doctors who traveled from the Eastern Roman Empire. Some of these doctors have been identified as Nestorian Christians. In 683, Emperor Gaozong had a headache and blindness, and his visual difficulties were successfully treated by Qin Minghe, who used needles on the emperor's head in two places. The doctor's name suggests that he was from Daqin, that is, the eastern Roman Empire, and some scholars identify him as a Nestorian missionary.[411]

Du Huan (735-812 CE) of China spent time in Arab regions as a prisoner of war. He noted in *Jingxing ji* (Notes on the Places Passed By):

> [The doctors of] the Eastern Roman Empire are good at treating eye diseases and diarrhoea. Some of them can predict disease before it comes. Some of them can carry out craniotomy to remove worms.[412]

In 831, Li Deyu went to Nanzhao in Yunnan Province to bring captives from Chengdu and Huayang back to Chengdu. Li Deyu noted that one of the captives was an eye doctor from Daqin.[413]

The Byzantine ophthalmic texts retained the language of the ancient Greeks, including the division of blinding conditions between *hypochyma*, the lighter *glaukos* eye, and the normal-appearing eye (amblyopia or amaurosis). The cleric Leo of Thessalonica (9th century) wrote that *hypochyseos* was an inflamed, thick liquid between the choroid and the cornea, which could be treated with *parakenteseos* (puncture). Leo cited Galen in this section. Glaucosis was an incurable transformation of the crystalline to a white color in the older patients. Leo also described *argemo* and *platykorias* (*i.e.* mydriasis).[414]

Lists of surgical tools that might have represented checklists for actual use in Byzantine hospitals include cataract-couching needles: *parcenteter* in a 9th-century manuscript and παρακεντέριος (*parakenterios*) in the 11th century.[415]

---

411 Li 2023.

412 Ming 2007. Li (2023) identifies doctor as coming from the area of Morocco, or a region southeast of Spain.

413 Li 2023.

414 Fronimopoulos, Lascaratos 1991, p. 369. From: Leonis Philosophi et Medici: Conspectus Medicinae. In: Leon 1840, chap. 25-35, pp. 140-147. Also known as: Leo Medicus, Leo the Physician, Leo Philosophus, Leo the Philosopher, Leo the Iatrosophist, or Leo the Mathematician. Lascaratos, Marketos 1991, p. 377. Lascaratos, Marketos 1988, p. 157.

415 Bliquez 1984, p. 187. 9th century: Codex Parisinus Latinus 11219; 11th century: Laurentianus gr. LXXIV 2.

The *Epitome* of Theophanes Chrysobalantes (fl. c. 950) stated that *hypochyma* was due to a coagulated fluid between the crystalline fluid and the choroid. Glaucoma was due to the crystalline fluid becoming *glaukos* (light colored) because of cold. No mention is made of any surgery, other than bloodletting, for any ophthalmic conditions. Theophanes also described *sclerophthalmia*, amblyopia, and amaurosis.[416]

Michael-Constantinos Psellos (c. 1017-c. 1078) wrote that glaucoma was an incurable change in the crystalline color, whereas *hypochyma* was from a moist formation between the cornea and crystalline. In *Carmen de re Medica*, he wrote that amaurosis produced blurred vision, whereas amblyopia involved confused vision. Psellos also mentioned mydriasis.[417]

The Jewish physician Symeon Seth (11th century) recommended fennel and partridge bile to treat amblyopia or early cataract. He also indicated that *sclerophthalmus* (a hard eye) is present in people who have difficulty discerning colors.[418] This observation appears novel.

In the 12th century, Stephanos of Tarsos, a resident in Constantinople of the Monastery of Saints Cosmas and Damian (the Cosmidian Monastery), was reported to have suffered from blindness for 5 years when the monastery doctors pierced and pricked his eyes with an iron instrument, returning his sight.[419] This may be the archbishop Stephanos of Tarsos, active at Antioch in 1135-1139.[420]

As described later, the 12th-century surgeon Theophilus of Constantinople taught Zacharias of Salerno and presumably was the source of Zachary's understanding about couching for *gutta kataracta*. The physician Nicolas Myrepsus (13th century) recommended collyria for glaucosis and eye cancers.[421] Nicolas probably spent time in Nicaea and Alexandria and compiled the texts of Galen.

The Sivas Hospital in Constantinople, founded in 1217, had oculists on its staff.

Johannes Zacharias Actuarius (c. 1275-c. 1328) agreed that *hypochyma* is curable, whereas glaucoma is not, because in the latter, the lens is destroyed by a foreign moisture. Amaurosis was a complete loss of vision without an observable cause,

---

416 Fronimopoulos, Lascaratos 1991, p. 369. Often called Theophanes Nonnus. Lascaratos 1998, p. 391.

417 Fronimopoulos, Lascaratos 1991, p. 369. Lascaratos 1998, p. 391. Lascaratos, Marketos 1988, p. 157.

418 Lascaratos 1998, p. 391.

419 Lascaratos 1992, p. 145.

420 Trial & deposition of Radulf of Domfront [in 1139]. http://db.pbw.kcl.ac.uk; Also written Stephan of Tarsus, archbishop in Antioch in 1135: Edbury, Phillips 2003, p. 41.

421 Lascaratos 1998, p. 391.

whereas amblyopia was due to obstruction of the optic nerves or the brain. Actuarius also mentioned *argema*, and mydriasis, which involved loss of vision.[422]

Ophthalmology continued to be written about after 1453 and the fall of Constantinople, now called Kostantiniyye. Amirdovlat Amasiatsi (1420-1496) was an Armenian doctor who trained in Amasia in the 1450s and had arrived in Constantinople by the end of the 1450s. He described cataract couching in detail:

> It is necessary to puncture eye tissues, and insert a needle, and drain the [indurated] cataracts, and then, the eye will clear up and be cleansed, and when you make sure that all of the [cataract] was drained, then lay a sleeping patient down on his back, put a plaster made of rose oil and egg yolk on his eyes, put a pillow under his head, and [secure the plaster with] a bandage. And let him remain in the dark room wearing the bandage for three days.[423]

Amasiati (1420-1496) was born in Amasia in about 1420 and trained in Amasia and Sebastia in the 1450s.[424] After Mohammed II captured Constantinople in 1453, he made Amirdovlat his chief eye surgeon (*charah-pashi ramatanin*).[425] Amirdovlat wrote his *Benefits of Medicine* in Philipopolis (current Plovdiv, Bulgaria) in 1469.[426]

In 1465, Serafeddin Sabuncuoglu (1385-1470 AD), who also practiced at the hospital at Amasia, wrote a surgical treatise in Turkish, which covered cataract surgery.[427]

---

422 Fronimopoulos, Lascaratos 1991, p. 369. Lascaratos 1998, p. 391. John Actuaris, De Diagnosi, Lib II, Ch. J'. Lascaratos, Marketos 1988, p. 157.

423 Vardanian 1999, p. 41. It is tempting to speculate that "draining" the cataract relates to cataract aspiration, but this translation is from Middle Armenian, to Russian, and then English, and so nothing conclusive could be stated without examination in the primary language. In addition, he does not describe an assistant applying suction. This passage is denoted [46:217] in the original work. Amasiati visited numerous other regions. He travelled around Macedonia in the late 1450s. He apparently travelled around Persia in the 1450s, as he frequently mentioned Shiraz, Khorasan, Gurgan, Isfahan, and Tabriz (Vardanian 1999, pp. 33, 88, 101).

424 Vardanian 1999, p. 143.

425 Vardanian 1999, pp. 33-34.

426 Vardanian 1999, p. 34.

427 Oguz 2004, p. 192.

## *Longshu pusa yanlun* (9th Century)

This Chinese treatise, translated as *Treatise of Bodhisattva Nagarjuna on Eye (Diseases),* is thought to date from the early 9th century.[428] The cataract method was as follows:

> The manifestation of cataract is very versatile. It can be divided morphologically into the following four types: (1) surface irregular or uneven type, (2) surface smooth type, (3) brittle ice type and (4) snow-white type. In addition to these four common types, some were classified as floating type or sinking type. Before learning to perform cataract surgery, the beginner should learn to identify properly which type of cataract the patient has and to grade the severity according to maturity. It is also important to differentiate the cataract as 'hot' type or 'cold' type. If it is the 'hot' type more than the 'cold' type, the patient should take the drug *ze-shih* to suppress the hotness before surgery. Otherwise, the patient will suffer from chest tightness after the operation. If the patient has 'empty heart' he will suffer from dizziness or be frightened after the operation. These patients should take *jen-shin wang, jin-ying gaw* or other similar medication according to the individual patient's condition.
>
> The manifestation of cataract ranges from mild to severe, and the needles used during the operation should be adjusted according to the severity of the cataract. Generally speaking, a small needle should be used in the mature cataract, and a large needle should be used in the premature cataract. The operative day chosen should be a sunny, windless day. The operator should calm down before the operation. The location where the needle enters the eyeball should be adjusted according to the laterality of the operative eye to avoid the nose. It will be difficult to perform the operation if the operator neglected the position of the nose.[429] Before the operation, the patient should face south. The operator should fix the eyeball to avoid rotation during the operation. After deciding the location to penetrate the eyeball, the needle should enter the eyeball slowly. The force should be proper. It should be applied lightly at first and become heavier after entering the eyeball. If the direction of the needle were deviated, the needle would damage intraocular tissues. If the needle damages the blood-ring, a severe hemorrhage would occur after the needle was removed from the eyeball.
>
> So it is important to remove the needle gently. If a hemorrhage did happen, the operator should compress the wound gently, or use hot steam to heat the wound. If a hemorrhage cannot be stopped by the above methods, the operation would fail. If the patient felt pain during the operation, the procedure should be stopped until

---

428 Mishima 2004, pp. 88-89; Deshpande, Fan 2012, pp. 108-112. Here we provide the translation from Mishima (2004).

429 Deshpande and Fan (2012, p. 110) have here: "Depending on the eye that is to be operated is left or right, the doctor should use his (left or right) hand. The needle is to enter at the small end. Operating the eye from the nose separation (internal canthus) is not very desirable."

the pain has disappeared. The needle should be entered to the pupil, and in that position, the needle should touch the lens and push it gently into the vitreous cavity. After that, the operator may ask the patient whether he can see better or not. If the patient has found his vision did improve, the operator should close the patient's eye and remove the needle. After removing the needle, the patient should keep quiet for a while, and the vision will improve afterward.

After the operation, the eye should be patched for seven days. The patient should lie down in a supine position. Other people should not talk loudly around the patient. The patient should be very careful when he sits up, leaves the bed, or performs any activity. The patient should not do any activity forcefully. During the postoperative month, the patient should not wash his face to avoid the dirty water contaminating the wound. The patient should avoid sexual behavior. He should avoid any irritating food. During the postoperative year, he should not eat wine-noodles. The eye patch can be removed after seven days. Although the patient can see better at that time, he will see some snow-like floating material. This symptom will improve gradually. The patient should not use his eyes too often in that period. If the patient complains of eye pain, it is a bad sign. After the postoperative fourteen days, the eye patch can be removed totally. If floaters still persist, the poorly healing wound caused it; the patient should avoid any harmful activity and leave enough time for the eye to recover during the postoperative three months.[430]

# Avoid Sex and Alcohol Postoperatively (9th Century)

Beginning in the 9th century, both Arabic and Chinese works advised the patient to avoid sex and alcohol postoperatively. The Syrian author Šim'ūn, whose fragments in al-Rāzī's *Continens* have been estimated to date from the mid-9th century, wrote the following about cataract:

Šim'ūn says: 'Couching (a cataract) is only indicated if the patient cannot see by night nor by day, and (if) he does not suffer from a headache or a cough; once (the cataract) is couched, (the patient) must lie still, like dead, not moving (at all), and he should avoid anger, sexual intercourse, and wine. In the early stage(s) of cataract let (the patient) snuff cocks' gall or infused saffron, or paint (his eyelids) with the water of wild pennyroyal or with (a salve made from) pepper and musk.'[431]

---

430 Mishima 2004, pp. 88-89.

431 Kahl 2015, pp. 44-46, 323. Celsus had required "abstinence" (abstinentia) postoperatively, by which he meant fasting (De Medicina 2.16). Antyllus forbid cataract patients from taking the "the wine of dates or vegetables" Sapientia Artis Medicinae proscribed drinking wine postoperatively. As noted in the previous section, , Longshu Pusa Yanlun of the 9th century had instructed: "The patient should avoid sexual behavior."(Mishima 2004, p. 88-89) The explicit prohibition against sex postoperatively might be present in the Ayurvedic works, but is harder to date. The vulgate edition of the Susruta Samhita noted in the 17th chapter of the Uttaratantra noted: "The disorder occurs by injury to head, physical exercise, coitus, vomiting, fainting and anger and also if punctured in too immature stage."(Susruta, Sharma

Similarly, Ammar of Cairo wrote in the 11th century that postoperatively, "The patient has to beware of light, candles, sexual intercourse, vomiting, crying and constipation for 40 days."[432]

We find in the Chinese literature that in the 9th century, *Treatise of Bodhisattva Nagarjuna on Eye (Diseases)* advised:

> The [postoperative] patient must not face the wind, or look at the sun and should abstain from sexual activities. He should be careful as regards abstinence rules. He should not eat five pungent substances, nor for one year should he drink excessively.[433]

Similarly, Nagarjuna's Comprehensive Treatise, mentioned in 1111 CE, advised for the postoperative patient:

> He should not have violent emotions or think of sexual activities. A husband and wife should have separate beds for a period of [one] hundred days. Face should not be washed for a month.[434]

---

2014, vol. 3, p. 206), or, alternatively, "A relapse of the deranged Dosha is caused by a blow on the head, physical exercise, sexual excesses, vomiting, epileptic fits, or by an act of piercing the Linga-nasa (cataract) during its partially developed (D. R. immature) stage."(Susruta, Bhishagratna 1916, vol. 3, p. 80) However, the prohibition against sexual activity postoperatively is not explicitly mentioned in the corresponding passage of the 878 Nepalese text of the Susruta Samhita, though restrictions relevant to use of oils must be followed (Birch, Wujastyk 2022). The 31st chapter of the Cikitsasthana of the Susruta Samhihta, on the use of sneha (unction/oils) does not mention sexual activity explicitly (Susruta, Sharma 2018, vol. 2, p. 552-565). This chapter does note: "The internal use of a Sneha is forbidden to persons suffering from ascites, fever, delirium, alcoholism, aversion to food and vomiting, as well as to weak, corpulent, thirsty, fatigued, or intoxicated persons."(Susruta, Bhishagratna 1911, vol. 2, p. 556) The injunction against sexual activity is not mentioned in the 17th chapter of the Uttarasthana of the Astanga Samgraha of Vagbhata (Vagbhata, Murthy 2000, vol. 3, p. 156). Emphasis on the importance of excessive indulgence in wine or women is found in the 25th chapter on Snehavidhi Adhyaya (oleation therapy) of the Sutrasthana of the Astanga Samgraha of Vagbhata (Vagbhata, Murthy 2003, vol. 1, pp. 432-447). The 14th chapter of the Uttarasthana of the Astanga Hrdayam of Vagbhata notes that postoperatively, the patient's "control is by (adopting) the regimen prescribed for sneha pana (chapter 16 of Sutrasthana)."(Vagbhata, Murthy 2017, vol. 3, p. 134) In the 16th chapter of the Sutrasthana of the Astanga Hrdayam of Vagbhata, on snehavidhi (oleation therapy), we read that it is used for those "who indulge more in wine, women, and exercise,...and...who are suffering from diseases of vata, ophthalmia, blindness..."(Vagbhata, Murthy 2016 vol. 1, p. 209), and that the patient "should use warm water only for all his activities, maintain celibacy...[avoid a] breeze..."(p. 214) See Chapter 3 on India..

432 Hirschberg, Lippert; Blodi et al. 1993, p. 164.

433 Deshpande, Fan 2012, p. 111. *Longshu pusa yanlun.*

434 Deshpande, Fan 2012, p. 141. *Longmu zong lun.*

## Dislocated Cataracts Resembling Mercury (11th Century)

Beginning in the 11th century, we find dislocated cataracts compared to mercury, because they are mobile. Ibn Isa of 11th-century Baghdad wrote:

> ...a cataract may look exactly like pure quicksilver, and on rotating the eyeball it may move quickly about like that substance.[435]

Khalifah al-Halabi of 13th-century Aleppo wrote about the "mercury-like cataract. It is bad and not suitable for surgery. Its cause: combination of a cold mixture of the brain and eye which condenses and becomes added to the fluid flowing towards the eye. Characteristic: it moves up and down in the hole in the iris like mercury."[436] In one manuscript, there is smaller print attributing this teaching to Galen, but another manuscript from Paris does not have this attribution.[437] In one of Khalifah's patients, the couched "cataract had risen again, revolving around the pupil like a top...The cataract floated between the cornea and the iris surrounding the pupil, moving like mercury."[438] The patient could see, so Khalifah did not intervene further.

The Chinese Nagarjuna's Comprehensive Treatise, mentioned in 1111 CE, describes:

> *Hua yi nei zhang*—An internal obstacle due to slippery screen...the brain fat flows downward, the liver *qi* rises up and strikes (the eye). In the pupil there is a screen resembling a pearl of mercury...It will be beneficial to turn it using a golden needle... Only (when you try to) open it (remove the screen using surgery), it becomes bigger and then suddenly smaller. It is similar to a mercury-pearl that moves. Although needling it is convenient, while taking out with a needle, it comes back to the original place.[439]

## The Spread of Couching toward the Periphery of Europe in the 12th Century

The Renaissance is said to have begun in Southern Europe in the 14th century. But some ophthalmic advances were made even earlier. Spectacles were invented in Italy in the late 13th century. Dissection was practiced in the 16th century, and the correct anterior location of the crystalline lens, which had been understood in antiquity, was rediscovered.[440]

---

435  Ibn Isa, Wood 1936, p. 177.
436  Blodi et al. 1993, p. 215.
437  Blodi et al. 1993, p. 226.
438  Blodi et al. 1993, pp. 219-220.
439  Deshpande, Fan 2012, p. 150. Treatise name *Longmu zong lun*.
440  Leffler, Schwartz 2020b; Leffler, Wainsztein 2016.

Cataract couching was once again described in Southern Europe beginning in the 11th and 12th centuries, apparently influenced by travelers from Arabic-speaking regions. The practice of cataract surgery subsequently spread toward the northern periphery of Europe. This process is demonstrated graphically with maps in a subsequent chapter. A narrative of the earliest identified oculists in each country illustrates this process.

*Countries bordering the Mediterranean* were some of the earliest to have documented oculists or cataract surgeons. In the late 12th century, Master Zacharias was not able to study ophthalmology in Salerno and, therefore, traveled to Constantinople for training before returning to Italy.[441]

A student of William Congenis (c. 1175-1225) observed an unsuccessful couching of cataract (*cataracta*) at Montpellier, France.[442] In 1253, Abraham of Aragon was invited to treat Alfonso de Poitiers in France. In 1284, the oculist Vidal Espeçero of Monson in Aragon was asked to treat a nobleman's wife. However, the oculist was kidnapped en route by the man who requested him and held for ransom at the castle of Monfulco.[443]

In 1330, Draga Slava (Draga the Slav), presumably from the area of present-day Croatia, was licensed in Venice to practice medicine, on the basis of *"laudabilis curis et experimentis factis de morbo podagrorum et oculorum"*.[444] Amirdovlat Amasiati traveled around Macedonia in the 1450s, and in 1469, he practiced in Philipopolis (current Plovdiv, Bulgaria).[445] In 1670, Evliya Celebi wrote that in the Albanian town of Elbasan, "there are 47 doctors and pulse takers...There are three eye doctors...There are quite a number of surgeons."

In *German-speaking regions*, oculists can be identified beginning in the 13th century. Judah ben Asher (1270-1349) was born in Cologne and had ocular troubles beginning at age 3 months.[446] At 3 years of age, he was treated by a woman who only worsened his condition. Then "a Jewess, a skilled oculist...treated me for about two months, and then died. Had she lived another month, I might have received my sight fully." He moved to France at age 13, and Toledo at age 28 years, and always had limited vision.[447]

---

441 Lascaratos 1998, p. 391. Hirschberg, Blodi 1985, vol. 2, pp. 254, 257. Name given as Magister Zacharias, Master Zacharias, Magistri Zacharie. Zacharias book, apparently published the year after Hirschberg wrote, was: Tractatus de passionibus oculorum: qui vocatur sisilacera: id est, secreta secretorum. Compilatus circa annos 1143-1180.

442 McVaugh 2001.

443 Shatzmiller 1994, p. 67.

444 Stefanutti 1961, pp. 101-102; Park 1998; Gabrić, Henc-Petrinović 1993.

445 Vardanian 1999, p. 34.

446 Abrahams 2006, p. 163.

447 Abrahams 2006, pp. 163-169.

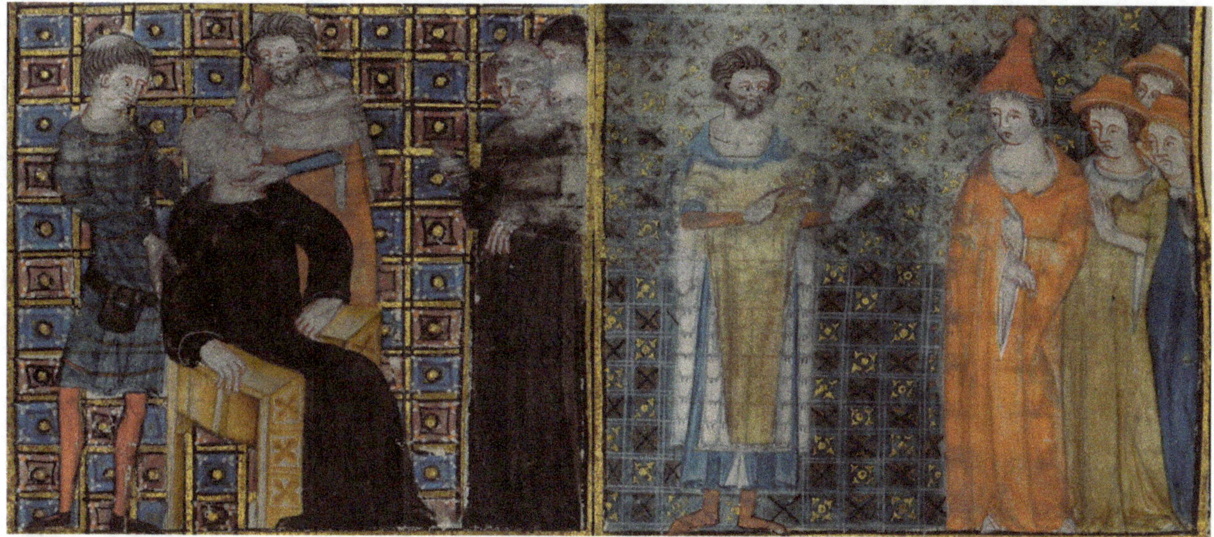

**Fig. 21.** Gilles le Muisit, abbot of St. Martin in Tournai, having a cataract couched by Master Jehan of Mainz in 1351.

In 1326, Princess Isabel, daughter of James II of Aragon, wrote to him from Graz indicating that she had a cataract (*"cateractam"*).[448] James II promised to send an ophthalmic specialist because the doctors in Graz were not very familiar with this condition, but James II died the next year before he could do this.[449] The oculist Jaume Roca of Aragon did travel to Graz to treat the princess in 1330, but she died before his arrival.[450]

In 1351, Master Jehan of Mainz passed through Tournai and couched the cataracts of Gilles le Muisit, abbot of St. Martin (Fig. 21).[451] Muisit wrote that he could then see "the sky, the sun, the moon, the stars," but could still not read or write.[452] As the abbot had to endure 3 years of complete blindness before the itinerant surgeon happened to arrive from central Germany, it is not clear that the procedure was well established in Tournai.[453]

In 1384, in Zurich, Meister Hans der Augenarzt was fined 9 schillings for beating a man in the street whom he accused of being a thief.[454]

---


448 McVaugh 2001.

449 McVaugh 2001.

450 Cardoner i Planas 1973, p. 174.

451 McVaugh 2001; Hirschberg, Blodi 1985, vol. 2, p. 258; Singer 2011, pp. 136-146.

452 McVaugh 2001.

453 Singer 2011, pp. 136-146.

454 Baas 1923.

In the British Isles, cataract surgeons appeared starting in the 16th century: Master Luke in London in 1562, "Maister Awin [a] Parisian" in Edinburgh in 1595, and William Read in Dublin in 1684.[455]

*Eastern Europe* had oculists in the 14th century. In the 1330s, a French doctor was summoned to Wroclaw to treat the eyes of King John of Bohemia.[456] When he proved incompetent, he was thrown into the Oder River. Then a Muslim practitioner was invited to treat the king's other eye at Prague and harmed other patients. The doctor had extracted a promise of safe conduct in advance. In 1339, the king traveled to Montpellier, where he was given medical treatment by Guy de Chauliac. The king returned blind to Prague and died at the Battle of Crecy.[457]

In the second half of the 14th century, Al-Shazilī (or Shadhilī) of Egypt described a Turkmen man in (presumably Southern) "Russia" (presumably near the location of the modern city of Odesa) and a Christian Russian in the Byzantine Empire who were familiar with the hollow needle for cataract aspiration.[458]

In 1469, a letter to the people of Bártfai (Bardejov) indicated that the oculist who was sent completely blinded the parish priest of Varanno in Slovakia with his bold cutting (*per suas scissuras*).[459]

In about 1471, a surgeon, Hans von Dockenburg (Her Johan von Tockenburgk), originally from the Swiss canton of Schwyz, successfully removed an arrow from the arm of King Matthias of Hungary.[460] It was said that the king had offered to handsomely reward anyone who could successfully remove the arrow, but had threatened death of the surgeon if the effort were unsuccessful. Dockenburg took up the challenge successfully, was granted a large fortune, and was knighted. As this healing by Toggenburg is not known from Hungarian sources, it is possible that Toggenburg invented the king's conditions in his subsequent writings. In his early days, Toggenburg practiced in Alsace. Toggenburg served King Matthias from about 1471 to 1474. Toggenburg advertised at the October fair in Leipzig in 1477 as "*De Cyrurgico et Oculista... Her* Johan von Tockenburgk."[461]

Guttmann Eberkard practiced as an oculist in Brasov, Romania, in 1615.[462]

*Along the Baltics*, oculists are found beginning in the 15th century. In 1400, three marks were given to an eye doctor (*ogenarczte*) who was sent by the grand master

---

455  Leffler et al. 2021.

456  McVaugh 2001.

457  McVaugh 2001.

458  Leffler, Samara, et al. 2020; Savage-Smith 2000.

459  Gyula 1929, p. 84. Town of Vranov nad Topľou, Slovakia.

460  Gyula 1929, p. 300.

461  Gyula 1929, pp. 297-300.

462  Gyula 1929, p. 86.

to King Vytautas of Lithuania.[463] In 1685, "Daniel Croon of Danzig, an oculist," was granted permission to erect a booth in the market square in Tallinn for 3 weeks, "providing that he does not miss the sermons."[464] In 1695, an itinerant oculist in Frankfurt boasted that he had obtained from an oculist friend in Riga a cataract needle that could extract cataracts.

In 1627, an "eye man" was listed on the staff of the Pharmaceutical Prikaz (Aptekarskiy Prikaz) in Moscow.[465] In 1630, the name David Broon (Brun) appears in Moscow as an oculist.[466] In 1631, his salary was 55r. He also received a horse and forage/allowance. In September 1644, he was the only oculist at the apothecary. He practiced as an oculist in Moscow until his death in 1651.[467] In 1630, Hans Johann Schultz's name appeared in Moscow as an oculist. In 1632, he served with the army. He was in Russia until 1644, when his vacant position was filled by Caspar Bartelov.[468]

*In Scandinavia*, oculists arrived beginning in the 15th century. In 1461, Kersten of Lübbeck, described as "mester Kersten, *de ogen arste*," had a debt to the town of Uelzen. In 1464, Kersten practiced in Randers in Jütland and was listed as buying oxen.[469] In 1465, Kersten still owed a debt for the purchase of 20 oxen.[470]

In 1589, David Heberlin, probably of Germany, was a *"Chirurgus et Ophthalmicus"* who settled in Telemark, Norway.[471]

In 1642, Steiner, known as the *"Danziger oculisten"*, made eye balms for Count Jakob de la Gardie (d. 1652), as his eyesight failed, at the Makalös Palace in Stockholm.[472] In 1771, regimental surgeon C. H. Deneke, assisted by Professor J. Haartman, performed a bilateral cataract extraction by the Daviel method in Helsinki. Deneke had studied with Olof af Acrel at Uppsala, and also in France, England, and Germany.[473]

*In the New World*, oculists arrived from the 17th century onward. In 1611, Francisco Drago of Genoa practiced in Mexico City.[474] In 1628, he was likely the oculist

---

463 Capaite 2013.

464 Kitching 1995.

465 Zimin 2018.

466 Unkovskaya 1999, p. 64; Zimin 2018.

467 Unkovskaya 1999, p. 64.

468 Unkovskaya 1999, p. 64.

469 Norn 2016, Baas 1923.

470 Marx 1970, p. 6.

471 Reichborn-Kjennerud et al. 1985, p. 140.

472 Axel-Nilsson 1984, pp. 40, 48.

473 Vannas 1984, p. 5.

474 Leffler, Wainsztein 2016.

who traveled from Mexico to Lima, Peru, to perform a cataract surgery.[475] In 1751, John Morphy performed a couching on Montserrat. In 1761, oculist William Stork began practicing in Philadelphia.

# Benevenutus Grassus (12th or 13th century)

Benevenutus Grassus authored *De Oculis*, an ophthalmic work influential well into the 17th century.[476] Grassus was an oculist and a teacher at Salerno and later Montpellier in the 12th or 13th century. He stated that he visited both hot and cold countries.[477] He was familiar with the language used in Arabic-speaking regions, as well as regions of Italy and Greece. He frequently invoked Jesus Christ, and he administered "Jerusalem pills" and described himself as "Benevenutus of Jerusalem."[478] Grassus' procedure for couching cataracts was used by oculists well into the 17th century throughout Europe:

> Having spoken of the characteristics and causes of the curable cataracts, let us consider their cure. In the first place, they cannot be entirely cured until they are complete [ripe] and properly formed.[479] The proof that this stage is reached is the patient's inability to see clearly the sun by day or the light of a candle by night…the trouble lies within the coats of the eye, especially the albugineus, and is the result of a disintegration of that humor so that a coagulated watery substance is poured out between the light and the crystalline humor. On this account both the Saracens and the Arabs call this form of cataract *linzaret*,[480] that is, fluid that has putrified in the eye. The doctors of the Salerno School give it a Latin name, *catharacta*, because the foul fluid has fallen down between the tunics and the light of the eye…A proper cure begins with a purgative, using my Jerusalem pills,[481] compounded only by me. The formula of these is spurge, half an ounce, hepatic aloes, five ounces, to be ground with sugar of roses. After purgation, at the third hour, the patient should be placed astraddle a bench, as if on horseback. Now be seated on the same bench face to face with the patient, who will keep one eye closed.[482] So begins the operation in the name of our Saviour Jesus Christ. With one hand raise the upper lid, and with the other hold a silver needle and direct it toward the outer lacrimal region. Then perforate the eye coats, pushing and turning the instrument around with the fingers until you touch the diseased matter, which the Saracens and Arabs call linzaret

---

475  de Trazegnies Granda 2012, pp. 98, 116, 244.

476  Leffler, Schwartz, Davenport, et al. 2014, p. 12.

477  Grapheus, Wood 1929, p. 27.

478  Grapheus, Wood 1929, pp. 75, 78-79.

479  *Nisi prius compleantur et bene firmentur* (Grapheus, Wood 1929, p. 32)

480  The Old French codes reads *illincosarar*, which Wood also surmises to be of Arabic origin (Grassus, Wood 1929, p. 33).

481  *Ieraclis* is in the Paris manuscript, which Wood surmises is an abbreviation of *hierosolimitantis*.

482  The *Compendil* manuscript has *both* eyes here (Grassus, Wood 1929, p. 33).

(but which we call cataract), with the point of the needle, and dislodge it from its position in front of the pupil. Then push it well below, holding it there until you have said four *pater nesters*. Then carefully and slowly turn the needle back to its first position in front of the eye. If the cataract follows the instrument and shows itself in front, you must again depress it, pushing it this time as much as possible towards the ear. Then withdraw the needle in the same manner that it was inserted…After the operation the patient's eye must be closed, and he should be kept in bed on his back in a shady part of the house. He must not be moved or allowed to look at a light for eight days, during which period the eye operated on must be dressed with white of egg twice a day and twice during the night. His diet should be soft, fresh eggs with bread…Finally, after eight or nine days, let the patient make the sign of the Cross and leave his bed. He may now bathe in cold water…The needle should be made of gold or silver. I am opposed to the use of steel…Take note, also, that a gold instrument especially clarifies objects with which it comes in contact because of its inherent power over cold and dampness.[483]

As with *Sapientia*, Grassus categorized cataracts as four curable and three incurable types.[484] Grassus explained that Arabic authors called this *linzaret*, which meant a putrefied water (*aqua*), but that at Salerno, they called it *cataractam*, "because the foul fluid has fallen down between the tunics and the light of the eye."[485] The curable cataracts [*cataractarum curabilium*][486] all began with the letter "c":

1) "White like the purest chalk" [*alba sicut calx purissima*] often caused by trauma,
2) "A white color but with a tendency to turn bluish" [*alba et assimilator colori celestino*], perhaps a celestial or sky color, caused by errors in diet,
3) Another "bluish white" associated with headache, that is *alba* with either (depending on the manuscript consulted) *cinericio*, which suggests gray, or *ceruleo*, which was an ambiguous blue or green eye color.[487] The description of a cataract as *ceruleo* echoes the ancient characterization of a suffusion as caerulean in the works of Celsus.
4) The fourth type of curable cataract has "a yellowish cast" [*cinericia citrina*] and is "the hardest of them all."[488]

---

483 Grapheus, Wood, 1929, pp. 32-34.

484 Grapheus, Wood 1929, pp. 31-32.

485 Grapheus, Wood 1929, p. 33. Latin from Grassus 1897, p. 19. Instead of *linzaret*, some manuscripts have *illincosarar* (Grapheus, Wood 1929, p. 33) or *elemeserat* (Grassus 1897, p. 19). It is unclear how any of these variants relate to the Arabic ophthalmic terms.

486 Grassus 1897, p. 23.

487 Grapheus, Wood 1929, p. 39. In Latin: Grassus 1897, p. 17. In the 1474 manuscript, the second curable cataract was *alba* with *celestrino* (Grassus 1474, p. 7). The third type of incurable cataract was *cinericio* in the 1897 edition, but *ceruleo* in the 1474 manuscript (p. 7).

488 Grapheus, Wood 1929, pp. 32, 36. In Latin: Grassus 1897, p. 17.

The three incurable types of cataract were *gutta serena*, the green pupil, and mydriasis. Grassus cited and was influenced by "Johannitus" (Hunain).[489] Grassus noted that Johannitus divided eye colors into four types: "black [*niger*], whitish [*subalbidus*] changeable colors [*varius*] and bluish-green [*glaucus*]," but Grassus himself felt the eye did not truly have any color—apparent color variation resulted from the manner and position at which the eye is viewed.[490] With respect to unfavorable cataract colors, Grassus made an important change. Constantine's translation of Johannitus identified *venetus* (Venice-blue) as the unfavorable pupillary color. In contrast, the only true color singled out by Grassus as incurable was green, *viriditas*.[491] The cataract has a "greenish color" [*quasi color viridis*] like a stone [*lapideo*]. The eye is bleared, there is sudden vision loss, there may be tearing, and it may be sequelae of pain or injury.[492]

Grassus' treatise was the first to lift the patient off the ground to be at the same height as the doctor. Interestingly, in the Chinese work *Essential Subtleties on the Silver Sea (Yinhai jingwei)* written between 1343 and 1373 AD, the doctor and patient also sit on a bench:

> The one should sit quietly to calm down one's own breath. Then one orders someone to bring a wooden bench, and one has a cotton quilt placed on it to allow for soft [sitting].[493]

In fact, just as Grassus did, the Chinese work also compares their posture to riding a horse:

> ...let the person sit facing (the doctor) as if riding a horse, so that he (the patient) is at the same level (as the doctor), neither high nor low.[494]

This posture is idiosyncratic, because the tradition since the works of Celsus and Suśruta had been for the doctor to be positioned higher than the patient.

Grassus was one of the first European authors to use a gold couching needle (though he also used a silver needle), and the Silver Sea text also recommended a golden needle.[495] The similarities between these texts despite wide geographic separation suggest that the Eastern and Western methods did not develop in complete isolation but could be influenced by both the same technological and cultural forces.

---

489  Grapheus, Wood 1929, pp. 28, 31.

490  Grapheus, Wood 1929, p. 28. Latin: Grassus 1897, p. 13.

491  Grassus 1474, p. 8.

492  Grapheus, Wood 1929, p. 39. In Latin: Grassus 1897, p. 25.

493  Kovacs, Unschuld 1998, p. 404.

494  Deshpande 2000.

495  Grapheus, Wood 1929, p. 33; Kovacs, Unschuld 1998, p. 404.

# The Silk Road Connection in Tabriz (1318)

One of the themes in this chapter is that ideas spread all along the Silk Road, from the Mediterranean to China (and perhaps in the other direction as well). In Tabriz, there was a hospital that might have facilitated this exchange of ideas. The hospital was built by Rashīd al-Dīn (c. 1247-1318), who had trained in medicine and became a minister in the Mongol administration. Rashīd al-Dīn hailed from a Jewish family but converted to Islam. His health facility in Tabriz, the Rab'-i Rashidi, was also called a "health house" (Dar-ush-Shafa) and had a medical school.[496] The staff included a physician, a surgeon, an oculist (*kaḥḥāl, jarrāḥ*), and two medical students.[497] The annual salary was 330 dinars for the physician, 100 dinars for the oculist, and 40 dinars for the pharmacist.[498] Two trainee-physicians (*mota ʿallem*) received a 30-dinar salary and were replaced every 5 years.[499] Students were also paid a 30-dinar salary.[500] The hospital housed 35 residents[501] and had procedural rooms.[502] Medical plants were grown in a garden.[503]

Rashīd al-Dīn tasked his foundation and hospital with spreading knowledge to students from as far away as Egypt, India, and China, as he described in a letter:

…The Rabe Rasidi [*i.e.* Rasidi Foundation] for the establishment and construction of which we had already made plans and preparations…is now completed. We have given dwellings to four hundred scholars, theologians, jurists and carriers of tradition, in the street which is named 'The Street of the Scholar'; daily payments, pensions, yearly clothing-allowances, soap-money, sweet-money have been granted for them all. We have established one thousand other students, who had come from all the possessions of Islam, in the hope of being educated under our protection, in the capital, Tabriz, and we have given orders for their pensions and daily pay to be granted from the tribune of Rum, Qostantiya [Istanbul] the Great, and Hindustan, in order that they may be comfortably and peacefully occupied in acquiring knowledge and profiting people by it.…Fifty skilled physicians who have come from the cities of Hindustan, China, Misr [Egypt], and Sam [Syria], have all been granted our particular attention and favour, in a thousand ways; we have ordered that they should frequent our 'House of Healing' [hospital] every day, and that every one should take ten students capable of learning medicine under his care and train them in the practice of this noble art. To each of the opticians and surgeons and bone setters, who work in and are attached to our hospital, we have ordered that five of the sons

---

496 Qajar 2005, p. 154.

497 Chipman 2007.

498 Chipman 2007.

499 Blair 2016.

500 Blair 2016.

501 Blair 2016.

502 Qajar 2005, pp. 154-156.

503 Qajar 2005, pp. 154-156.

> of our servitors should be entrusted so as to be instructed in the oculist's art, in surgery and manipulative surgery...[504]

According to one account, 500 teachers and 6000 students attended the facility for free (over an unspecified period of time).[505] The library had 600,000 books. In addition to surgeons, the hospital had oculists (*Khekhali*).[506]

## The Spread of Couching in Africa (1653)

The spread of cataract couching in the medieval and modern periods might provide clues about where couching originated. Cataract couching probably spread throughout Northern Africa in antiquity.

In the modern period, couching has been described farther south than the Mediterranean coast of Africa. In 1653, a patient traveled from Dienné to Timbuktu where he was successfully operated on for cataract.[507] Cataract surgery was also performed in Darfur in the 19th century.[508] In the modern period, cataract couching by traditional healers is found primarily in the regions of North Africa, spreading downward into the same areas where Islam had spread: Nigeria, Sudan, and so on.[509] The fact that couching has not traditionally been practiced in the more Southern areas of Africa, such as the Congo, could suggest that couching arrived in conjunction with Islam, and, in any event, probably did not start well South of the Sahara. For instance, if couching had started in areas of modern-day Nigeria, then it probably would have moved Southward with the waves of Bantu migration in the Common Era.

## A South Pacific Anomaly (2006)

One anomaly could call into question the single-origin theory of cataract couching. In a paper on cataract surgery in Papua New Guinea, we read that one 52-year-old woman had bilateral couching performed by a "traditionalist."[510] Upon inquiry with the authors, we learn that cataract couching in the country is not known on the main island of Papua, but occurs by traditional healers in Bougainville, in the Solomon Islands.[511] This is believed to be a traditional healing technique, rather than a skill taught to the islanders by Westerners. Bougainville is 6,500 km (4,000 miles) from Myanmar along the peninsulas and archipelagos of Thailand, Malaysia,

---

504 Taylor 1939, pp. 39-40.

505 Qajar 2005, pp. 154-156.

506 Qajar 2005, pp. 154-156.

507 Es-Sa'di, Houdas 1909, p. 445.

508 Al-Tunisi, Davies 2018, p. 171.

509 Crichton-Harris 2009, p. 311.

510 Garap 2006.

511 Personal communication, Garry Brian, 2019.

Indonesia, and Papua, in which we could not find evidence of couching. Whether couching arrived by a wayward traveler or whether it originated de novo in Bougainville is unknown.

# Conclusions

Close to 1500 BCE, in the Bronze Age, there are hints that cataract surgery might have been performed in Egypt or in Babylon, but none of the evidence from this period is definitive. Egyptian gods restored an eye, and venesection was performed close to the eye in Babylonia.

The evidence that cataract couching originated in Egypt is as strong as for any other region. The ancient Greek author pseudo-Galen suggested an Egyptian origin. There was enough time for cataract surgery to develop along the Nile, to be (possibly) sought by Cyrus of Persia in the 6th century BCE, to be discovered by the Greeks with the founding of Alexandria in 331 BCE, to be mentioned by Chrysippus of Soli in the 3rd century BCE, to be carried to Taxila by the Persians before Alexander the Great (or by the ambidextrous Greeks afterward), and then to be described in the *Suśrutasaṃhitā* in India in the early Common Era. A Mediterranean origin is suggested by the emphasis on ambidexterity.

Some ancient Greco-Roman ideas about cataract couching appeared in medieval Arabic successors, but did not spread eastward in time to be found in Ayurvedic treatises, or in early medieval Chinese works: the importance of the rough surface of the posterior iris, the needle entering an empty space, intentional discission, comparison of the couchable lesion with a goat's eye, preoperative pharmacologic mydriasis, using the same paracentesis site for reoperations, hypopyon drainage, placing metallic rings around the couching needle shaft, and possibly cataract extraction by aspiration. Covering the nonoperative eye eventually spread from the Mediterranean eastward into India and Tibet, but not during this early period.

Similarities between ancient Eastern and Western descriptions of cataract couching suggest that the procedure originated once and then spread throughout the world. It is possible to interpret many of the similarities as the Eastward spread of ideas, which originated close to the Mediterranean. Early Greek and Sanskrit descriptions of cataract couching both involve comparison of some cataracts to glass; colored entoptic phenomena; a preference for patients of intermediate ages; phlegm (or *kapha*) as a cause of couchable cataracts; the requirement for maturity of the cataract; pars plana puncture with avoidance of the blood vessels; perception of "flies, hairs, webs, and circles" with cataracts; central cataracts causing double vision; blowing on the eye; placing cotton on the eye; rubbing the eye; use of iron and silver instruments; turning the eyes toward the nose; and belief that an overly hard cataract was unsuitable for couching. In ancient Greece and India, the words for a healthy blue eye (*glaukos* and *nīla*, respectively) were also used to characterize an eye with poor vision, which could not be cured by surgery. In both Greek and

Indian works, the crystalline lens was compared to a lentil, and colored entoptic phenomena were described.

Some ideas were found along the Mediterranean, in the early Ayurvedic works of India, and in China: ambidexterity of the surgeon, use of copper or bronze needles, having the patient sitting outside, the favorable prognosis of pupil responses, and immediate vision testing.

Some ideas are found in the Greco-Roman works and later East Asian works, but not in the Ayurvedic works of India. The origin of cataracts from a fluid that descends from the brain; the treatment of cataracts with carp gall; comparison of cataracts to ice, snow, silver, or (when dislocated) mercury; performance of surgery on a warm day; preoperative marking of the site with a second instrument (or the instrument's handle); and (possibly) intentional discission fall all into this category. Presumably, these ideas were transmitted along the Silk Road orally, or in Indian works, which have not survived to our era, or the ideas were transmitted directly by Nestorian travelers to China. The demonstration of idea transfer along the Silk Road is consistent with other work demonstrating parallels between Hippocratic and Chinese anatomy and treatments presumably predating the Hippocratic era.[512]

In the area from the Mediterranean to Mesopotamia, we see a great deal of ophthalmic innovation. In addition to cataract couching with a solid needle, soft cataracts were intentionally divided in Greco-Roman practice. As we will see in a subsequent chapter, the medieval Arabic authors (and possibly the ancient Antyllus) described cataract aspiration by suction through a tube. Removal of a cataract by an inferior corneal incision is briefly alluded to in Greco-Roman antiquity and in the medieval period, but the descriptions are not detailed enough to exclude the possibility that a hypopyon was being drained.

# References


Abrahams I. *Hebrew Ethical Wills*. Philadelphia: Jewish Publication Society; 2006.

Aelian, Scholfield AF (trans.). *On the Characteristics of Animals*. Vol. II. Cambridge: Harvard University Press; 1959: 120-121.

Aelian, Scholfield AF (trans.) *On the Characteristics of Animals*. Vol. III. Books XII-XVII. Cambridge: Harvard University Press; 1959: 158-159.

Aëtius of Amida, Waugh RL (trans.). *The Ophthalmology of Aëtius of Amida*. Oostende: Wayenborgh; 2000: 85-86.

Albucasis, Spink MS, Lewis GL (trans.). *Albucasis on Surgery and Instruments: Abu al-Qasim Khalaf Ibn Abbas al-Zahrawi*. Berkeley: University of California Press; 1973: 252-256.

Al Safi A. *Traditional Sudanese Medicine: a Primer for Health Care Providers, Researchers, and Students*. Khartoum: al Safi; 2006: 156-395.


---

512  Craik 2009.

al-Tunisi M, Davies H (trans.). *In Darfur: An Account of the Sultanate and Its People, Volume Two*. New York: New York University Press; 2018: 171.

Aristotle, Taylor T (trans.). *On the Generation of Animals. The Treatises of Aristotle*. London: Robert Wilks; 1808: 421-423. Available from: books.google.com

Aristotle, Peck AL (trans.). *Aristotle Vol. XIII. Generation of Animals*. Loeb Classical Library Number 366. Cambridge: Harvard University Press; 1943: 492-499. https://archive.org/stream/generationofanim00arisuoft#page/n3/mode/2up

Ascaso FJ, Lizana J, Cristóbal JA. Cataract surgery in ancient Egypt. *J Cataract Refract Surg*. 2009;35:607-608.

Axel-Nilsson G. *Makalös: fältherren greve Jakob de la Gardies hus i Stockholm*. Kommitten for Stockholmsforskning; 1984.

Baas K. Augenärztliches aus dem späteren deutschen Mittelalter. *Albrecht von Graefes Archiv für Ophthalmologie*. 1923 Mar;111(1):84-90.

Baker P. Roman medical instruments: archaeological interpretations of their possible "non-functional" uses. *Soc Hist Med*. 2004;17:3-21.

Baker P. Collyrium Stamps: An Indicator of Regional Practices in Roman Gaul. *Eur J Archaeol*. 2011;14:158-189.

Bakhouche B. Calcidius' Theory of Vision between Geometry, Medicine, and Philosophy. *Revue dhistoire des sciences*. 2013;66(1):5-31.

Balaguer V. *História de Cataluña y de la Corona de Aragon*, Vol. 3. Barcelona: Librería de Salvador Manero; 1862: 608.

Bartisch G, Blanchard DL (trans.). *Ophthalmodouleia: That is the Service of the Eyes 1583*. Ostend: Wayenborgh, 1996:50-52.

Beckwith CI. *Greek Buddha. Pyrrho's Encounter with Early Buddhism in Central Asia*. Princeton: Princeton University Press; 2015: 8-113.

Beiram MMO. Traditional and folk medicines in ophthalmology. *Sudan Med J*. 1971;9:161-166.

Berrey M. Chrysippus of Cnidus: medical doxography and Hellenistic monarchies. *Greek Roman Byz Stud*. 2014;54:420-443.

Blair SS. Rab'-E Rašidi. *Encyclopædia Iranica*. 2016. iranicaonline.org

Bliquez LJ. Two lists of Greek surgical instruments and the state of surgery in Byzantine times. Dumbarton Oaks Papers, Vol. 38, *Symposium on Byzantine Medicine*, 1984:187-204.

Blodi FC, Rademaker WJ, Rademaker G, et al. *The Arabian Ophthalmologists. Compiled from original texts by J. Hirschberg, J. Lippert, and E. Mittwoch*. Riyadh: King Abdulaziz City for Science and Technology; 1993: 152-302.

Blomstedt P. Cataract surgery in ancient Egypt. *J Cataract Refract Surg*. 2014;40:485-489.

Boutell C. *The Handbook to English Heraldry*. 11th ed. London: Reeves & Turner. 1914: 35-37.

Breton P. On the native mode of couching. *Transact Med Phys Soc Calcutta*. 1826:341-382.

Čapaitė R. The Topic of health in the letters of Grand Duke Vytautas of Lithuania and his contemporaries. *Lithuanian Hist Stud*. 2013 Jan 8;18(1):1-45.

Cardoner i Planas A. *Historia de la medicina a la Corona d'Arago* (1162-1479). Barcelona: Scentia; 1973: 174-176.

Carvalho AS. *História da Oftalmologia Portuguesa: até ao m do século XVI*. Lisboa: Boletim da Sociedade de Oftalmologia. 1939;Tomo I:16-34.

Celsus, Spencer WG (trans.). *On Medicine. Books I-IV*. Volume I. Loeb Classical Library 292. Cambridge, MA: Harvard University; 1935: 154-155.

Celsus, Spencer WG (trans.). *De Medicina*. Vol. II. Cambridge, MA: Harvard University Press; 1938: 62-222.

Chipman L. Islamic pharmacy in the Mamlūk and Mongol realms: Theory and practice. *Asian Med.* 2007 Oct 16;3(2):265-278.

Cobo J, Martínez Vidal À. *La práctica médico-quirúrgica en la primera generación del movimiento" novator" a través de las obras de Juan Bautista Juanini* (Milán, 1632-Madrid, 1691). Universitat Autonoma de Barcelona. 2004.

Collins K. Jewish physicians and the Porguguese Medical Diaspora. *Vesalius* 2020;XXVI(1):91-106.

Cotter W. *Miracles in Greco-Roman antiquity: A sourcebook for the study of New Testament miracle stories*. Routledge; 2012.

Craik EM. Hippocratic bodily "channels" and oriental parallels. *Med Hist.* 2009 Jan;53(1):105-116.

Crichton-Harris A. *Poison in small measure: Dr. Christopherson and the cure for bilharzia*. Leiden: Brill; 2009: 311.

de Trazegnies Granda L. *Sevilla y la Lima de Pizarro-Ensayo histórico*. Sevilla: Bubok; 2012:98,116,244.

DeGaris Davies N. *Two Ramesside Tombs at Thebes*. New York: Metropolitan Museum of Art; 1927: 69-Plate XXXVII.

Demaitre L. *Medieval Medicine: the Art of Healing from Head to Toe*. Santa Barbara, CA: Praeger; 2013: 165.

Deshpande V. Indian Influences on Early Chinese Ophthalmology: Glaucoma as a Case Study. *Bull Sch Orient Afr Stud.* 1999;62:306-322.

Deshpande V. Ophthalmic surgery: a chapter in the history of Sino-Indian medical contacts. *Bull Sch Orient Afr Stud.* 2000;63:370-388.

Deshpande VJ, Fan KW. *Restoring the Dragon's Vision. Nagarjuna and Medieval Chinese Ophthalmology*. Hong Kong: City University of Hong Kong, 2012:88.

Diogenes Laertius. Hicks RD (trans.). *Lives of Eminent Philosophers*, Vol. I. Books 1-5. Loeb Classical Library 184. Cambridge: Harvard University Press, 1925:440-443.

Dioscorides, Osbaldeston TA, Wood RPA (trans.). *de Material Medica…in Modern English*. Johannesburg: Ibidis; 2000.

Dunglison R. *A Dictionary of Medical Science*. Sixth ed. Philadelphia: Lea and Blanchard; 1846: 25.

Ebeigbe JA. Traditional eye medicine practice in Benin-City, Nigeria. *South African Optometrist* 2013;72:167-172.

Edbury PW, Phillips J. *The Experience of Crusading, Volume 2: Defining the Crusader Kingdom*. New York: Cambridge University Press; 2003.

Edge C, Gibbins D. Underwater discovery of Roman surgical equipment. *BMJ* 1988;297:1645-1646.

Elgood C. *Safavid medical practice: or, the practice of medicine, surgery and gynaecology in Persia between 1500 AD and 1750 AD*. London: Luzac; 1970.

Elliot R. *The Indian Operation of Couching for Cataract*. New York: Hoeber; 1918: 14.

Es-Sa'di, Houdas O (trans.). *Tarikh es-Soudan par Abderrahman ben Abdallah ben 'Imran ben 'Amir es-Sa'di. Traduit de l'Arabe par O. Houdas*. Paris: Leroux; 1909: 445-446.

Fan (Ka Wai). Couching for cataract and Sino-Indian medical exchange from the sixth to the twelfth century ad. *Clin Exp Ophthalmol.* 2005 Apr;33(2):188-190.

Feugère M, Künzl E, Weisser U. Les aiguilles à cataract de Montbellet (Saône-et-Loire). Contribution à l'étude de l'ophtalmologie antique et Islamique. Die starnadeln von Montbellet (Saône-et-Loire). Ein beitrag zur antiken und Islamischen augenheilkunde. *Jarbuch des Römisch-Germanischen Zentralmuseums Mainz* 1985;32:24-508.

Fischer KD. Die Klappe fällt—frühe Belege für lat. Cataracta als Bezeichnung einer Augenkrankheit. *Medizinhistorisches Journal*, Bd. 35, H. 2 (2000):127-147.

Fried LS. Cyrus the Messiah? The historical background to Isaiah 45: 1. *Harv Theol Rev*. 2002 Oct;95(4):373-393.

Friedenwald J, Morrison S. The history of the enema with some notes on related procedures (Part I). *Bull Hist Med*. 1940;8:68-114.

Fronimopoulos J, Lascaratos J. The terms glaucoma and cataract in the ancient Greek and Byzantine writers. *Documenta ophthalmologica* 1991;77(4):369-375.

Gabrić N, Henc-Petrinović L. A brief review of the development of ophthalmology in Croatia. *Acta Medica Croatica: Casopis Hravatske Akademije Medicinskih Znanosti*. 1993 Jan 1;47(1):1-4.

Galen, Duckworth WLH, Lyons MC, Towers B. *Galen on anatomical procedures: the later books*. New York: Cambridge University Press; 2010: 31.

Galen, Johnston I (trans.). *Galen. On Diseases and Symptoms*. Cambridge: Cambridge University Press, 2006: 211-215.

Galen, Johnston I, Horsley GHR (trans.). *Method of Medicine*, Volume II, Books 5-9 2011. Cambridge, MA: Harvard University Press; 2011: 398-399.

Galien [Galen], Kühn KG (éd.). *Introductio Seu Medicus. Galeni opera omnia*. vol. 14. Leipzig: Car. Cnoblochii, 1827: 675. www.biusante.parisdescartes.fr Accessed February 23, 2020.

Garap JN, Sheeladevi S, Brian G, et al. Cataract and its surgery in Papua New Guinea. *Clin Exp Ophthalmol* 2006;34:880-885.

Geller MJ. *Ancient Babylonian Medicine: Theory and Practice*. Oxford: Wiley-Blackwell; 2010: 58-184.

Gibbins DJ. The Roman wreck of c. AD 200 at Plemmirio, near Siracusa (Sicily): second interim report: The domestic assemblage 1: medical equipment and pottery lamps. *Int J Naut Archaeol*. 1989;18:1-25.

González Arce JD. Los proyectos de ordenanzas generates de médicos, cirujanos y boticarios de Castilla (ca. 1491-1513). *Dynamis*. 2011;31(1):207-226.

Gordon BL. Ophthalmology in the Bible and in the Talmud. *Arch Ophthalmol*. 1933;9(5):751-788.

Grant RL. Antyllus and his medical works. *Bull Hist Med* 1960;34:154-174.

Grant RL. Antyllus, the elusive surgical genius of antiquity: an analysis of his writings. *Surgery* 1961;50:572-578.

Grapheus B [Grassus], Wood CA (trans.). *De Oculis Eorumque Egritudinibus Et Curis*. Stanford: Stanford University Press; 1929: 33-148.

Grassus [Grapheus] B. *L'Opera oftalmojatrica di Benvenuto nei codici negli incunabuli e nelle edizioni moderne*. Modena: Societa Tipografica; 1897. https://archive.org/stream/loperaoftalmoja00grapgoog#page /n101/mode/2up

Grassus B. *De oculis eorumque aegritudinibus et curis*. Ferrara, 1474, p. 8. Available at: http://gallica .bnf.fr/ark:/12148/bpt6k58490t/f14.image.r=.langEN

Grayson M, Keates RH. *Manual of Diseases of the Cornea*. Boston: Little Brown; 1969: 277-279.

Gregory of Tours. *Grégoire de Tours: Histoire des Francs; livres I-VI. Texte du Manuscrit de Corbie*. Paris: Henri Omont; 1886: 152.

Grisar H. *Il Sancta Sanctorum ed il suo tesoro sacro: scoperte e studii dell'autore nella Cappella Palatina lateranense del medio evo*. Roma: Civiltà Cattolica; 1907: 160.

Grzybowski A, Ascaso FJ. Indirect evidence of cataract surgery in ancient Egypt. *J Cataract Refract Surg*. 2014;40:1944-1945.

Gyula Magyary-Kossa. *Magyar orvosi emlékek. Értekezések a magyar orvostörténelem köréből 2. A Magyar Orvosi Könyvkiadó Társulat Könyvtára 122*. Budapest: Kotet, 1929. Available from: https:// library.hungaricana.hu/hu/view/KlasszikusOrvosiKonyvek_153

Hamilton M. *Incubation: Or, the Cure of Disease in Pagan Temples and Christian Churches*. London: Henderson; 1906: 13-18.

Hassel FJ, Künzl E. Ein römisches Arztgrab des 3. Jahrhunderts n. Chr. aus Kleinasien. *Medizinhist J* 1980;15:403-421.

Heuzé V, Tran G, Eugène M, et al. *Babul (Acacia nilotica) 2016.* Accessed January 18, 2020. Available online: https://agritrop.cirad.fr/582523/1/ID582523.pdf

Heymans H. Eine Hülse mit Arztinstrumenten aus Maaseik (Belgien). *Archäologisches Korrespondenzblatt* 1979;9:97-100.

Heymans H, Janssens P., De. "Trousse d'Oculiste" van Maaseik. *Hades* 1975-76;14-15:10-12.

Hibbs VA. Roman surgical and medical instruments from La Cañada Honda (Gandul). *Archivo Español de Arqueología* 2018;64:111-134.

Hippocrates of Cos, Potter P (trans.). *Hippocrates V, Affections. Diseases 1. Diseases 2. Loeb Classical Library 472.* Cambridge, MA: Harvard University Press; 1988: 170-291.

Hippocrates, Potter P (trans.). *Hippocrates. Vol. VIII. Places in Man. Glands. Fleshes. Prorrhetic 1-2. Physician. Use of Liquids. Ulcers. Haemorrhoids and Fistulas.* Loeb Classical Library 482. Cambridge: Harvard University Press; 1995: 154-261.

Hippocrates, Potter P (trans.). Sight. In: *Hippocrates Vol. IX. Loeb Classical Library 509. Coan Prenotions. Sight. Anatomical and Minor Clinical Writings.* Cambridge, MA: 2010; 154-155.

Hirschberg J. Die Bruchstücke der Augenheilkunde des Demosthenes. *Archiv für Geschichte der Medizin.* 1919 May 1(H. 3/4):183-188.

Hirschberg J, Blodi FC (trans.). *The History of Ophthalmology. Vol. 1. Antiquity.* Bonn: Wayenborgh Verlag; 1982: 34-349.

Hirschberg J, Blodi FC (trans.). *The History of Ophthalmology. Volume Two. The Middle Ages;the Sixteenth and Seventeenth Centuries.* Bonn: Wayenborgh Verlag; 1985: 41-685.

Holth S. *Greco-Roman and Arabic bronze instruments and their medico-surgical use. Videnskapsselskapets Skrifter. I. I. Maternatisk-Naturvidenskabelig.* No. 1. Klasse, Kristiana, 1919:3-20.

Holth S. An Arabic bronze needle from antiquity for depression of cataract. *Br J Ophthalmol.* 1924;8:266-268.

Hossfeld FL, Zenger E (trans.), Maloney LM (trans.), Baltzer K (ed.). *Psalms 3: a commentary on Psalms 101-150.* Minneapolis: Fortress Press; 2011: 608-617.

Hunain Ibn Is-Haq (Johannitus), Meyerhof M (trans.). *The Book of the Ten Treatises on the Eye Ascribed to Hunain Ibn Is-Haq (809-877 A.D.).* Cairo: Government Press; 1928: 122.

[ibn Isa] 'Alī ibn 'Īsá Kaḥḥāl, Wood CA. *Memorandum Book of a tenth-century oculist for the use of modern ophthalmologists.* Northwestern University; 1936: 165-187.

[ibn Sina] Abu Ali al-Husayn ibn Abd Allah ibn Sina (Avicenna), Sardo PA (trans.). Bakhtiar L (ed.). *The Canon of Medicine (al-Qanun fi'l-tibb) (The Law of Natural Healing). Volume 3. Special Pathologies.* Chicago: Kazi Publications; 2014: 207-274.

Jackson R. A set of Roman medical instruments from Italy. *Britannia* 1986;17:267-271.

Januensis S (Simon de Gênes). *Clavis sanationis.* Patavina. 1474. Archive.org.

Jouanna J, Allies N (trans.). Egyptian Medicine and Greek Medicine. In: *Greek Medicine from Hippocrates to Galen: Selected Papers.* Leiden: Brill; 2012: 15-16.

Kahl O. *The Sanskrit, Syriac and Persian sources in the Comprehensive book of Rhazes.* Leiden: Brill; 2015: 44-46.

Kitching LP. New land for research: The German-language theater in Reval/Tallinn and Hans Jacob Wigandt's petition of 1630. *Journal of Baltic Studies.* 1995 Mar 1;26(1):25-44.

Konczacki JM, Aterman K. Regina Salomea pilsztynowa, ophthalmologist in 18th-century Poland. *Surv Ophthalmol.* 2002 Mar 1;47(2):189-195.

Koren N. *Jewish physicians: a biographical index.* Jerusalem: Israel University Press; 1973.

Kovacs J, Unschuld PU. *Essential Subtleties on the Silver Sea. The Yin-hai jing-wei: a Chinese Classic on Ophthalmology*. Berkeley: University of California Press; 1998: 4-211.

Künzl E. *Medizinische Instrumente aus Sepulkralfunden der Römischen Kaiserzeit*. Cologne: Rheinland Verlag GmbH; 1983: 12-114.

Lang ML. War and the rape-motif, or why did Cambyses invade Egypt? *Proceedings of the American Philosophical Society*. 1972 Oct 13;116(5):410-414.

Lascaratos J, Marketos S. A historical outline of Greek ophthalmology from the Hellenistic period up to the establishment of the first universities. *Documenta Ophthalmologica* 1988; 68:157-169.

Lascaratos J, Marketos S. Ophthalmological therapy in hospitals (xenones) in Byzantium. *Documenta ophthalmologica*. 1991;77(4):377-383.

Lascaratos J. Miraculous ophthalmological therapies in Byzantium. *Documenta Ophthalmologica*. 1992;81(1):145-152.

Lascaratos J. Ophthalmology in Byzantium (10th-15th centuries). Medicina Nei Secoli. Arte e Scienza. *J History Medicine*. 1998;11(2):391-403.

Leffler CT. Ophthalmic Healing in the Bible: New Insights and Analysis. Sep. 2022. researchgate.net

Leffler CT, Schwartz SG, Davenport B, et al. Enduring influence of Elizabethan ophthalmic texts of the 1580s: Bailey, Grassus, and Guillemeau. *Open Ophthalmol J*. 2014;8:12-18.

Leffler CT, Schwartz SG, Davenport B. Congenital cataract surgery during the early enlightenment period and the Stepkins oculists. *JAMA Ophthalmol*. 2014;132:883-884.

Leffler CT, Schwartz SG, Hadi TM, et al. The early history of glaucoma: the glaucous eye (800 BC to 1050 AD). *Clin Ophthalmol*. 2015;9:207-215.

Leffler CT, Schwartz SG, Giliberti FM, et al. What was Glaucoma Called Before the 20th Century? *Ophthalmol Eye Dis*. 2015;7:21-33.

Leffler CT, Hadi TM, Udupa A, et al. A medieval fallacy: the crystalline lens in the center of the eye. *Clin Ophthalmol*. 2016;10:649-662.

Leffler CT, Wainsztein RD. The first cataract surgeons in Latin America: 1611-1830. *Clin Ophthalmol* (Auckland, NZ). 2016;10:679.

Leffler CT, Schwartz SG, Wainsztein RD, et al. Ophthalmology in North America: Early Stories (1491-1801). *Ophthalmol Eye Dis* 2017;9:1179172117721902.

Leffler CT, Schwartz SG, Peterson E, et al. Cataract couching and the goat's eye. *Acta Ophthalmol*. 2018;96:755-756.

Leffler CT, Klebanov A, Samara WA, et al. The history of cataract surgery: from couching to phacoemulsification. *Annals of Translational Medicine*. 2020 Nov;8(22).

Leffler CT, Schwartz SG. Glaucoma in the ancient Greek and Roman worlds. In: Leffler CT (ed.), *The History of Glaucoma*. Oostende: Kugler/Wayenborgh; 2020a:1-46.

Leffler CT, Schwartz SG. Glaucoma during the Enlightenment and Early Modern Periods (1700-1849). In: Leffler CT (ed.), *The History of Glaucoma*. Oostende: Kugler/Wayenborgh; 2020b:145-196.

Leffler CT, Samara WA, Hadi TM, et al. *Glaucoma in the Medieval Arabic World. The History of Glaucoma*. Oostende: Kugler/Wayenborgh; 2020: Apr 17:47-74.

Leffler CT, Schwartz SG, Peterson E, et al. The first cataract surgeons in the British Isles. *Am J Ophthalmol*. 2021 Oct 1;230:75-122.

Léon (philosophe). Anecdota medica graeca e codicibus mss. *Lugduni Batavorum: apud S. et J. Luchtmans*. 1840: 140-147. archive.org

Lev E. *Jewish Medical Practitioners in the Medieval Muslim World*. Edinburgh University Press; 2021.

Leverett FP. *A New and Copious Lexicon of the Latin Language*. Boston: Wilkins, 1837: 95.

Li W. Seeing the Light Again: A Study of Buddhist Ophthalmology in the Tang Dynasty. *Religions*. 2023 Jul 7;14(7):880.

Liddell HG, Scott R. αἰγίς. In: *A Greek-English Lexicon*. Oxford: Clarendon Press; 1940. www.perseus. tufts.edu

Lind LR. *Studies in Pre-Vesalian Anatomy: Biography, Translations, Documents*. Philadelphia: American Philosophical Society; 1975: 70.

Livy (Titus Livius), Moore FG. *History of Rome*, Volume VII: Books 26-27. Loeb Classical Library Num. 367. Cambridge: Harvard University Press; 1943: 324-325.

Longrigg J. Anatomy in Alexandria in the Third Century B.C. *Br J Hist Sci*. 1988;21:455-488.

Lucian, Macleod MD (trans.). *Lucian. Vol. VII. Dialogues of the Gods*. Cambridge: Harvard University Press; 2015: 264-265.

Lucretius Carus T, Leonard WE (trans.). *On the Nature of Things*. London: Dent; 1921: 147.

Magnus H, Waugh RL. *Ophthalmology of the Ancients (in Two Parts). Part 1*. Oostende: Wayenborgh; 1998: 95.

Marganne MH. *Inventaire analytique des papyrus grecs de médecine*. Genève: Droz, 1981: 7-267.

Marganne MH. *L'ophtalmologie dans l'Egypte gréco-romaine d'après les papyrus littéraires grecs*. New York: E.J. Brill; 1994: 120-121.

Márquez de Aracena R. The "mistress of healing eyes" in 15th century Spain. *Israel Med Assoc J: IMAJ*. 2012 Jul 1;14(7):465-466.

Marx R. *Geschichte der Augenheilkunde in Lubeck*. Lubeck: Akademie Lubeck; 1970.

Maximus of Tyre. Trapp MB (trans.), *The Philosophical Orations*. Translated by M. B. Trapp. Oxford: Clarendon Press; 1997: 87.

Maxwell-Stuart PG. *Studies in Greek Colour Terminology. Vol 1. Glaukos*. Leiden: Brill Archive; 1981: 26-165.

Maxwell-Stuart PG. *Studies in Greek Colour Terminology: Vol 2. Charopos*. Leiden: Brill; 1981: 4-5.

McEvilley T. *The Shape of Ancient Thought. Comparative Studies in Greek and Indian Philosophy*. New York: Allworth Press; 2002: 1-450.

McVaugh MR. Cataracts and hernias: aspects of surgical practice in the fourteenth century. *Med Hist*. 2001 Jul;45(3):319-340.

Meulenbeld GJ. *A History of Indian Medical Literature. Vol. IA. Text*. Groningen: Forsten; 1999: 303-651.

Meyer-Steineg T. *Die Starnadel aus Kos. Chirurgische Instrumente des Altertums*. Jena: Fischer; 1912: 45.

Meyerhof M. L'operation de la cataracte du Chirurgien Antylle d'Alexandrie. In: Koumaris J (ed.), *Livre d'or à l'occasion du jubilé de vingt-cinq ans d'activité chirurgicale du docteur Théodore L. Papayoan-nou ... Le Caire, le 8 mai 1932*. Naumburg-Saale: Lippert & Co; 1932: 115-119.

Milne JS. *Surgical Instruments in Greek and Roman Times*. Oxford: Clarendon Press; 1907: 69-176.

Ming C. The transmission of foreign medicine via the silk roads in Medieval China: A case study of Haiyao Bencao. *Asian Med*. 2007 Oct 16;3(2):241-264.

Mishima S. *The history of ophthalmology in Japan*. Oostende: Wayenborgh; 2004: 64-89.

Moulherat C, Tengberg M, Haquet JF, et al. First evidence of cotton at Neolithic Mehrgarh, Pakistan: analysis of mineralized fibres from a copper bead. *J Archaeol Sci*. 2002;29:1393-1401.

Naqvi NH. Surgical instruments in the Taxila Museum. *Med Hist*. 2003;47:89-98.

Neale M. *Madhyamaka and Pyrrhonism. Doctrinal, Linguistic and Historical Parallels and Interactions between Madhyamaka Buddhism & Hellenic Pyrrhonism*. Regent's Park College, University of Oxford. DPhil; August 2014.

Nene YL. Indian pulses through the millennia. *Asian Agri-History* 2006;10:179-202.

No author listed. *Digital Corpus of Sanskrit. Suśrutasaṃhitā*. Su, Utt. 17, 64.1. Available online: http://www.sanskrit-linguistics.org/dcs/index.php?contents=texte&PhraseID=12476 Accessed January 9, 2020.

Norn M. Danish Ophthalmology—from start to 1865. *Acta Ophthalmologica*. 2016 Mar;94(2):205-209.

Oguz H, San I, Verit A, et al. Ophthalmic techniques described by Serefeddin Sabuncuoğlu (1385-1468 AD). *Clin Exp Ophthalmol*. 2004;32(2):192-195.

Pansier, P. Collectio Ophtalmologica Veterum Auctorum. Paris: Baillière, 1903-1908.

Park K. Stones, bones and hernias: Surgical specialists in fourteenth-and fifteenth-century Italy. In: *Medicine from the Black Death to the French Disease*. Routledge; 1998: 110-130.

Paton WR, Tueller MA (trans.). *The Greek Anthology. Vol. 1. Books 1-5*. Cambridge: Harvard University Press; 2014: 100-101.

Paton WR (trans.). *The Greek Anthology, Volume III: Book 9: The Declamatory Epigrams*. New York: Putnam; 1917: 64-65.

Paulus Aegineta. Adams F (trans.). *The Seven Books of Paulus Aegineta: Translated from the Greek*. Vol. 2. London: Sydenham Society; 1846: 279-280.

Paulus Aegineta, Libri V-VII. Heiberg JL (editor), *Corp. Med. Graec. IX 2*. Leipzig et Berlin; 1924: 59-61. http://cmg.bbaw.de/epubl/online/cmg_09_02.php

Philostratus, Conybeare FC (trans.). *Philostratus: the Life of Apollonius of Tyana. The Epistles of Apollonius and the Treatise of Eusebius*. With an English Translation by F. C. Conybeare, MA. In Two Volumes. I. London: Heinemann; 1912.

Pi HT. A brief historical sketch of native ophthalmology in China. *Nat Med J China* 1929;15:604-618.

Pilsztynowa RS, Roczniak W (trans.). *My life's travels and adventures: an eighteenth-century oculist in the Ottoman Empire and the European hinterland*. New York: Iter Press; 2021: 75.

Pliny, Bostock J, Riley HT. *The Natural History of Pliny*. Vol. V. London: Bell; 1900: 137.

Pliny, Rackham (trans.). *Natural History, Volume II: Books 3-7*. Loeb Classical Library 352. Cambridge; 1940: 516-519.

Praxagoras, Steckerl F (trans.). *The Fragments of Praxagoras of Cos and His School*. Leiden: Brill; 1958: 73-75.

Priaulx OD. Art. III.—The Indian Travels of Apollonius of Tyana. *J Roy Asiat Soc*. 1860 Jan;17:70-105.

Qajar C. *The Famous Sons of Ancient and Medieval Azerbaijan*. 2005. Available from: http://elibrary.bsu.edu.az/files/books_460/N_363.pdf Accessed April 10, 2022.

Rambo VC. Couching operation in Tibet. *AMA Arch Ophthalmol*. 1955;54:471-473.

Reggiani Massarini AM. Indagini sui materiali dell'Antiquario del Museo Nazionale Romano. *Archaeologia Laziale* 1988;9:455-466.

Reichborn-Kjennerud I, Grøn Fr, Kobro I. *Medisinens historie i Norge*. Grøndahl & Søns Forlag; 1936. New Edition, Kildeforlaget Oslo; 1985: 140-141.

[Rhazes] Abū Bakr Muḥammad ibn Zakarīyā Rāzī. Faraj ben Salim (trans.). *Continens Rasis*. Venice: Johannes Hamman; 1529: 41. Available online: https://www.wdl.org/en/item/9553/view/1/102/ Accessed January 20, 2020.

Robinson ML, Lovicu FJ. The lens: historical and comparative perspectives. In: Robinson ML, Lovicu FJ (eds.), *Development of the Ocular Lens*. Cambridge University Press; 2004: 5-273.

Ruben Maslatón S. *Historia de los judíos de España y Portugal: situacón social, política y religiosa; basándose en textos de José Amador de los Ríos; posee apéndice al final de la obra*. Mexico: Jerusalem de Mexico; 2014.

Savage-Smith E. Hellenistic and Byzantine ophthalmology: trachoma and sequelae. *Dumbarton Oaks Papers*. 1984;38:169-186.

Savage-Smith E. The practice of surgery in Islamic lands: myth and reality. *Soc Hist Med*. 2000;13(2):307-321.

Sextus Empiricus, Bury RG (trans.). *Sextus Empiricus. Volume I. Outlines of Pyrrhonism*. Loeb Classical Library 273. Cambridge, MA: Harvard University Press; 1933: 28-29.

Shastid TH. History of ophthalmology. In: Wood CA, ed. *The American Encyclopedia and Dictionary of Ophthalmology*. Vol. XI. Chicago: Cleveland Press; 1917: 8580-8669.

Shatzmiller J. *Jews, Medicine, and Medieval Society*. Berkeley, CA: University of California Press; 1994.

Simplicius of Cilicia. Kalbfleisch C. ed. *Commentaria in Aristotelem Graeca. Vol. VIII. Simplicii in Aristotelis Categorias Commentarium*. Berlin: Reimeri; 1907: 401.

Simplicius of Cilicia. Gaskin R (trans.). *Simplicius: on Aristotle categories 9-15*. London: Bloomsbury Academic; 2013: 143.

Singer J. *Blindness and therapy in late medieval French and Italian poetry*. Boydell & Brewer; 2011: 136-146.

Stefanutti U. *Documentazioni cronologiche per la storia della medicina, chirurgia e farmacia in Venezia: dal 1258 al 1332*. Venezia: Ferdinando Ongania Editore; 1961.

Strabo, Jones HL (trans.). *Geography, Volume II. Books 3-5*. Cambridge: Harvard University Press; 2015: 126-127.

Sushruta, Bhishagratna KKL (trans.). *An English Translation of the Sushruta Samhita. Vol. I. Sutrasthanam*. Bose: Bhaduri; 1907: 257.

Sushruta, Bhishagratna KKL (trans.). *An English Translation of the Sushruta Samhita. Vol. III. Uttara-Tantra*. Calcutta: Bhaduri; 1916: 25-79.

Suśruta, Birch J, Wujastyk D. *A Translation of the New Edition of the Suśrutasaṃhitā*. Susruta Project website; 2021. Available from: https://sushrutaproject.org/ Accessed July 10, 2021.

Susruta, Sharma PV. *Suśruta-saṃhitā. With English translation of text and Dalhana's commentary along with critical notes. Vol. I. (Sūtrasthanā)*. Varanasi: Chaukhambha Visvabharati; 2018: 61-275.

Suśruta, Sharma PV. *Suśruta-saṃhitā. With English translation of text and Dalhana's commentary along with critical notes. Vol. III. (Kalpasthana and Uttaratantra)*. Varanasi: Chaukhambha Visvabharati; 2014: 141-619.

Taylor OE. *Architecture of Northwest Persia Under the Il-Khan Mongols*. PhD Thesis. University of Chicago; 1939: 39-40.

Terrada ML. Las prácticas médicas extraacadémicas en la ciudad de Valencia durante los siglos XVI y XVII. *Dynamis: Acta Hispanica ad Medicinae Scientiarumque Historiam Illustrandam*. 2002;22:85-120.

Theophilus of Antioch. Grant RM (trans.). *Theophilus of Antioch ad Autolycum*. Oxford: Clarendon Press; 1970: 4-11.

Theophrastus. Hort AF (trans.). *Enquiry into Plants. Vol. I. Books 1-5*. Loeb Classical Library 70. Cambridge, MA: Harvard University Press; 1916: 470-471.

Tontchéva G. Découvertes de tombes d'Odessos. *Bulletin de la Société Archéologique à Varna* 1961;12:39-40.

Torres Fontes J. Los médicos murcianos en el siglo XV. *Miscelánea Medieval Murciana*. 1973;(1):240-267.

Triplett K. *Buddhism and medicine in Japan: a topical survey (500-1600 CE) of a complex relationship*. Walter de Gruyter GmbH & Co KG; 2019 Nov 18.

Unkovskaya MV. *Brief Lives: a Handbook of Medical Practitioners in Muscovy, 1620-1701*. London: Wellcome Institute. 1999: 64.

[Usaybia] 'Uṣaybi'a, Kopf L (trans.), Plessner M (ed.). *Ibn Abī 'Uṣaybi'a. History of Physicians*. Translated for the National Library of Medicine, Bethesda (1971). Printed in Jerusalem; 2017: 48, 490.

Vāgbhata, Srikantha Murthy KR (trans.). *Aṣṭāṅga-saṃgraha. Vol. III. Uttarasthāna*. 2nd ed. Varanasi: Chaukhambha Orientalia; 2000:133-155.

Vāgbhata, Srikantha Murthy KR (trans.). *Vāgbhaṭa's Aṣṭāñga Hṛdayam. Vol. III (Uttara Sthana)*. Varanasi: Chowkhamba Press; 2017: 133.

Vannas S. *History of Ophthalmology in Finland*. University of Helsinki; 1984.

Vardanian SA. *Amirdovlat Amasiatsi: A Fifteenth-century Armenian Natural Historian and Physician*. Academic Resources Corp; 1999.

Vegetius Renatus, Publius Flavius. *Pub. Vegetij viri illustris Mulomedicina*. Basileae: Petrum Pernam; 1574.

Vegetius Renatus, Publius Flavius. *Vegetius Renatus of the Distempers of Horses, and of the Art of Curing Them*. London: Millar; 1748.

Von Staden H. *Herophilus—The Art of Medicine in Early Alexandria*. Cambridge: Cambridge University Press; 1989:20-578.

Wallis F. *Medieval Medicine: A Reader*. Toronto: University of Toronto Press; 2010: 17-57.

Wlaschky M. Sapientia artis medicinae: ein fruhmittelalterliches Kompendium der Mediczin. In: HE Sigerist (ed.), *Kyklos*. Leipzig: Thieme, Verlag, Institut fur Geschichte der Medizin; 1928: 103-113.

Zimin I, Grzybowski A. Spectacles in Russia from Moscow Tsardom to Russian Empire. XVII–first half of the XIX Century. *Archiwum Historii i Filozofii Medycyny*. 2018(81):92-99.

# 2. The Ophthalmology of the Hellenistic Surgeon Antyllus

Mathias Witt, MA, MD, PhD[1]

## Section 1: An Introduction to Antyllus

The ophthalmological fragments from book 1 of the lost surgical manual *cheirourgoúmena* (*Surgical Matters*) by the surgeon Antyllus (approximately 2nd century AD) constitute important sources for ancient eye surgery.[2] *Cheirourgoúmena* was a title common for surgical manuals in Hellenistic times. Authors like Leonides (1st century AD), Archigenes (1st/2nd century AD), and Heliodorus (1st/2nd century AD) who belonged, like Antyllus, to the Pneumatic school of medicine wrote such treatises. This group of physicians is, therefore, referred to as the "pneumatic surgeons," a term coined by Max Wellmann (1895). Of all these manuals, only fragments are preserved. Antyllus' *cheirourgoúmena* are the only ones of which not only Greek but also Arabic fragments have come down to us.

The title of Antyllus' *cheirourgoúmena* is only known from Greek, not from Arabic sources. The manual was arranged from head to toe and consisted of two parts. Part 1 included chapters on surgical procedures from the head to the abdomen, and part 2 covered surgeries on the urogenital system and possibly also proctologic operations. As opposed to other interventions, a considerable amount of text passages on ophthalmology, from book 1 of this surgical manual, are preserved as excerpts in Greek and Arabic sources. The fact that Antyllus' ophthalmological chapters were particularly cherished is proven by a testimony from Ḫalīfa from Aleppo (approximately 1256 AD), who does not refer to Antyllus by name, but simply by calling him "the Greek ophthalmologist" (see fragment 10 on the cataract below). The Byzantine medical compiler Aëtius of Amida (6th century AD) who usually draws his surgical passages from the more conservative and less innovative surgeon Leonides does not rely on him, when it comes to eye diseases, but on Antyllus.

---

1 Priv.-Doz. Dr. med. habil. Dipl.-Jur. Univ. Mathias Witt M.A., Institut für Ethik, Geschichte und Theorie der Medizin, Lessingstraße 2, 80336 München. E-mail: mathias.witt@med. uni-muenchen.de.

2 A scholarly edition with critical apparatus, translation, and commentary of all surviving fragments of this work is forthcoming (Witt [forthcoming-a]). The present chapter is an abridged and slightly modified excerpt of this publication, translated into English. All translations into English are mine.

## Elements of Antyllus' Biography

The surgeon Antyllus is an enigmatic figure. Although he enjoyed a certain fame in antiquity and Byzantine times, nothing certain is known about his biography. Thus, we neither know his date of birth, his education, course of studies, teachers, the place(s) where he lived, nor when and where he died. Even a rough chronological placement seems difficult. Antyllus is thought to have lived between the 1st and 4th centuries AD,[3] with the 2nd century AD being favored by scholars. The 4th century AD can at any rate be considered the *terminus ante quem*, since the Byzantine compiler Oribasius (325-403 AD) excerpted from Antyllus. The 1st century AD is, on the other hand, assumed to be the *terminus post quem*, because Antyllus seems to refer to the physician Archigenes (second half of the 1st century AD until the first half of the 2nd century AD) in a fragment of his treatise "On Therapeutical Aids," transmitted by Oribasius (Coll. med. 9,23,18-19). It is, however, questionable how conclusive this reference is. The mention of Archigenes does not necessarily have to go back to Antyllus himself, but could have been added by Oribasius who is known to juxtapose diverging opinions of different authors just the way this reference does. In other fragments of his works, Antyllus seems to refer to Hippocrates (twice) and to a certain Timocrates.[4] Nothing is known about Timocrates either, except for the fact that he must have been contemporary or before Galen who quotes a recipe by him (XII,887,K). It can even not be proven whether Galen (129-216 AD) knew Antyllus. Max Wellmann[5] affirms this with reference to Galen's commentary on the Hippocratic treatise "On Liquids." In this commentary, passages can be found that are elsewhere (by Oribasius) labeled as Antyllus excerpts. However, the commentary turned out to be a Renaissance forgery[6] so that Wellmann's argument is not valid any more. We, therefore, lack evidence of any Antyllus reception by Galen.

In any case, the sources indicate that Antyllus was perceived as an eminent surgeon. This is what we read in Paulus (6.33, chapter "On Laryngotomy"): "The best surgeons also described this operation. Thus Antyllus says: ..." In the glossary of a certain Cyrillus (5th century AD), lists of the most important representatives of various professional groups (historians, philosophers, poets) are given. Antyllus figures in the "list of excellent physicians," along with 18 prominent doctors, such as Hippocrates, Galen, and Diocles.

Although it is known, through a passage by the Roman poet Juvenal (Satire 6.366-373), that the surgeon Heliodorus lived in Rome and, through a passage in the pseudo-Galenic "Introduction," that Leonides was active in Alexandria (Ps.-Gal., Introd. IV 3, XIV,684,8seq. K.: Leōnídēs ho Alexandreús), Antyllus' local assignment to Alexandria can only be made with caution.

---

3  See Grant (1960) p. 155.

4  Aëtius 3.23, Oribasius Coll. med. 6,31,5seq. and Paul of Aegina 7,24,12.

5  Wellmann (1894), col. 2644 and Wellmann (1895), p. 104.

6  Ihm (2002), p. 106.

In Arabic authors, Antyllus is occasionally referred to as an "Alexandrian." In the *Kitāb al-Ḥāwī by al-Rāzī* (*ca. 865, † ca. 925 AD), the "therapy of the Alexandrian Antyllus" (*'ilāǧ Anṭīlis al-'Iskandarī*) is mentioned in a fragment on eyelid inflammation (see later in this chapter). In Ibn Abī Uṣaibi'a (*after 1194, † 1270 AD) (I, 109), Antyllus appears within a list of physicians who lived in the Alexandrian period. This list is, however, not necessarily reliable; a certain Sindahašār is also mentioned therein. This is not a personal name, but the corrupted Indian book titled *Siddhasāra*, a work by the Indian physician Ravigupta, who lived around 650 AD. Furthermore, we do not know exactly what Arabic authors meant by "Alexandrian." The term does not necessarily seem to refer to the city of Alexandria but to some kind of local affiliation with Alexandria or the Alexandrian school of medicine. For the Arabs, someone was likely to be "Alexandrian" who lived in the Alexandrian period, that is, the time when Egypt was not yet Islamized.

Some internal evidence with biographical relevance can, however, be retrieved from Antyllus' fragments: In a surgical fragment on tongue ankylosis (Orib. Coll. med. 45,16; CMG VI 2,1, 169seq.), Antyllus refers to the fact that Egyptians and Syrians have an unarticulated speech (presumably as Greek foreign speakers). This argument may suggest that Antyllus was a Greek native speaker himself and it might be a geographical hint to Alexandria. Had Antyllus lived in Rome or some other place of the Roman Empire, he might not have mentioned Egyptians and Syrians and expected his readers to follow his argument. In the same chapter on tongue ankylosis, Antyllus alludes to the fact that, in his time, the sounds of the Greek letters phi (φ) and chi (χ) were still pronounced plosively ([pʰ] and [kʰ]), rather than as fricatives, as in late antiquity and still in modern Greek ([f] and [ç]). This observation is, however, not suitable as a precise dating aid, since plosive pronunciation of these letters was still common in Egypt in the 2nd and 3rd centuries AD and the exact point of time, when the change in pronunciation took place, is unknown[7] (and is even likely to have been gradual rather than abrupt). In another surgical Antyllus fragment on atheromas (Orib. Coll. med. 45.5; CMG VI 2,1, 163, scholion to ln. 26), there is an etymological hint to, once again, Egypt: "The content of an atheroma resembles to what is called 'athera' by the Egyptians. They hereby designate a boiled mash made from white wheat flour." This remark could derive either from Antyllus' own linguistic experience in Egypt or simply from an etymological handbook. The latter is, however, quite likely since it is evident through text comparisons that the pneumatic surgeons like Leonides, Heliodorus, and Antyllus drew etymologies and definitions from a common etymological source, as I demonstrated elsewhere.[8]

Antyllus' individual writing style shows a self-confident and strong personality. Whereas Leonides and Heliodorus use a more neutral and objective style with impersonal formulations or verbs in the third person, Antyllus uses the first-person singular or plural. He repeatedly distances himself from his predecessors,

---

7 Allen, 1987, p. 23.

8 Witt (forthcoming-b).

providing his own judgments or statements ("The older surgeons did ... but we ..."), which is not known from any other ancient surgical author. Antyllus is usually counted among the "pneumatic surgeons" who adhered to the Pneumatic school of medicine, as stated earlier. However, he seems to have been eclectic to a certain degree, since, in his writing, elements of humoral pathology and of the methodist school of medicine can be found as well.[9]

## Ophthalmological Fragments

Ophthalmological fragments of the following chapters of Antyllus' surgical manual are transmitted in Greek and Arabic sources: "On Cataract," "On Trichiasis," "On Eyelid Inflammation/Loss of Eyelashes," "On Ectropion," "On Hydatid Cysts," "On Pterygium," and "On Tumors and Fistulas of the Eye" (*aigilops/anchilops*). The Arabic Antyllus fragments are mostly unedited (a critical edition is forthcoming).[10] The fragments on ophthalmology will be collected and presented here for the first time in English translation.

The majority of the Arabic Antyllus fragments are from the *Kitāb al-Ḥāwī fī al-ṭibb* by the Persian physician and polymath Abū Bakr Muḥammad ibn Zakariyyāʾ al-Rāzī (approximately 864-925 AD). *Kitāb al-Ḥāwī* is not a polished work, but a rather chaotic posthumous collection of excerpts Rāzī took throughout his life, with some of them being fairly verbatim and some free paraphrases or scattered remarks. There are repetitions and double passages throughout this work. In her fundamental study, Ursula Weisser (1991) developed a classification of excerpts in the Ḥāwī according to the degree of literalness. She distinguishes between four types of excerpts. This classification is also used in the following to characterize individual excerpts. The types are as follows:

Type 1: Quotations in the strict sense, text reproductions close to the original wording, at most short gaps

Type 2: Paraphrases, shortened excerpts, occasionally the sequence of arguments being changed

Type 3: Extensive passages, summarized in a few sentences

Type 4: Isolated statements, removed from their original context

No critical edition of the Ḥāwī exists so far, only a preliminary and incomplete one of the Arabic text that appeared in Hyderabad, India, from 1955 to 1971. There is also a medieval Latin translation that helps to fill gaps in the Arabic print edition since it is based on a better and more complete manuscript.

---

9  Grant (1960) p. 159seqq.

10  See fn. 1.

# Section 2: Antyllus on Pathologies of the Eyelid and of the Eye

This section covers Antyllus' account of all ocular pathologies, except for the numerous fragments on cataracts and cataract surgery, which are discussed separately in the next section. All of the following fragments have (more or less evident) parallels with the respective chapters on eye surgery in Paul of Aegina's book 6. These chapters in Paul can be identified as (more or less abridged) Antyllus excerpts with the help of parallel Arabic fragments, as discussed in more detail in the commentary sections. The Arabic Antyllus fragments offer surplus text in many instances, which supplements Paul's abridged excerpts and thus helps to get a better insight into how Antyllus' ophthalmological chapters might have originally looked like. In Paul, the sequence of chapters on eye pathologies is as follows:

6.12 On Ectropion, 6.13 On *Anabrochosmós* [Trichiasis Operation], 6.14 On Hydatid Cysts, 6.18 On Pterygium, 6.21 On Cataract, 6.22 On Aigilops.

Usually, Byzantine compilers like Paul of Aegina preserve, more or less, the order of chapters of the sources they excerpted from. One may, therefore, assume that Antyllus' sequence of chapters is reflected in Paul. Therefore, the fragments of Antyllus' ophthalmological chapters are, in the following, presented in Paul's sequence. Chapters that are not preserved in Greek but only in Arabic fragments ("Eyelid Inflammation/Loss of Eyelashes," *anchilops*) were incorporated into the sequence, where it seemed most appropriate.

**On Ectropion: Commentary**

Antyllus' chapter on the surgical treatment of ectropion (ie, pathologically everted eyelids) is only preserved in Greek (in Aëtius of Amida). No Arabic fragments on this topic can be found.

The operation described to correct lower eyelid ectropia consists of a tightening procedure after a wedge excision of tissue. Antyllus remarks at the end of the chapter that neither the ectropion of the upper eyelid can be cured nor that of the lower eyelid caused by paralysis (Bell's palsy) or excessive excision during surgery. The same applies to ectropion caused by extensive scarring, for example, as a result of ulcers or carbuncles. Antyllus adds that ectropion can be the result of a tumor in the corner of the eye (*aigilops* and *anchilops* tumors; see later for more on these).

A chapter on ectropion is also preserved in Paul of Aegina (6.12), which, however, has only few scattered verbatim parallels with the respective chapter in Aëtius. There is no complete sentence in parallel. Antyllus was certainly used by Paul (or his source), but heavily rephrased and abbreviated. Paul's chapter is, therefore, not counted as an Antyllus fragment and is not translated here.

**On Ectropion: Translation**

**Translation from the Greek of Aëtius of Amida, Libri medicinales 7.74 (ed. Olivieri, 1950 [CMG]).**

Antyllus' surgical treatment of ectropion

The larger excessive flesh formations have to be cut out with a scalpel, then to be treated with pulverized burnt copper or aloe with incense granules, and then to be treated the same way, after using fomentations. On the third day, you have to use honey after the steam bath until the aftertreatment starts. But if the ectropion is larger, you have to proceed as follows:
Starting from the outer part of the eyelid, you have to make two incisions in the shape of the letter lambda, where the narrow part is at the bottom, towards the cheek, and the wide one at the top, near the eyelashes. Then you have to cut out the lambda-shaped strips along with the underlying flesh, because the lower eyelid is not cartilaginous. The skin, however, must be kept intact. Then you have to connect the wound margins of the excised area with a suture. One suture made at the parts towards the eyelashes will be enough. This is how the eyelid will be brought into a curved shape and convex towards the inner parts. But if, for some reason, a scar developed on the outside of the eyelid, turning the eyelid outwards, you have to remove the lambda-shaped strip from the outer parts of the eyelid, as described. But do not cut very deeply, and unite the wound margins of the incision with a suture, as described. Then we stretch the scar with a hook from outside and stitch a needle with a double linen thread under the excessive flesh formation, throughout the entire scar, starting from the small [= temporal] corner of the eye, piercing the needle towards the large [= nasal] corner. If the needle is then placed [in the tissue], we push the linen thread down under both its ends and, by its help, stretch all of the excessive flesh upwards and thus carry out the excision, bringing out the excessive flesh together with the needle that has been inserted. After the surgical treatment, however, we fill the external opening with compresses and apply a twice folded one wetted with cold water; then, we put a bandage on and leave the folded compress in place, moistening it with cold [water] until the third day. But on the third day, we loosen it by wiping it off with warm water, with a sponge, because a steam bath will not help in these. For you have to be careful that the internal adhesion does not fail somehow. But after the threads have fallen off from them because the structures have grown together, it is safe to do a steam bath. You have to use it so that the scar becomes more tender and that the eye is relieved. Then you have to anoint the inside of the eyelid with astringent collyria. The external separation, however, must be maintained open throughout the entire treatment using fairly soft medicines. As a result of the yielding of the outer skin, the contraction will be of a certain size, in order to turn the eyelid inwards. But if an ectropion of the eyelid is caused by a tumor in the corner of the eye, then you will return the eyelid to its natural position by removing the tumor in the corner of the eye. But you should know that the ectropion of the upper eyelid cannot be cured. Furthermore, the one cannot be cured that is caused by a paralysis of the lower eyelid, equally the one caused by cutting out a stripe that is too broad, especially in the *catarrhaphé* operation [an operation that consists of suturing the eyelid downwards], and the one caused by a wide scar, when an ulceration has preceded, as is the case of carbuncles.

## On Trichiasis/*Anabrochismós*

This chapter deals with the surgical treatment of trichiasis using a thread loop. Trichiasis is a disease in which the eyelashes are pathologically turned inwards and rub against the cornea. The cause is an inverted eyelid (ectropion) or a double row of eyelashes (distichiasis). This surgical technique described by Antyllus is called *anabrochismós* (lit. "pulling up with a loop") in Greek. It was known under the name "illaqueation" in modern medicine (from Latin *laqueus,* which means loop), until the middle of the 20th century. Four fragments of this chapter have survived in Arabic, two of them in Rāzī's Ḥāwī.

## Fragment 1 on Trichiasis: Commentary

A comparison of Rāzī's Arabic with ʿAlī ibn ʿĪsā shows that both texts go back to the same source, that is, Antyllus. A similar chapter on *anabrochismós* is anonymously transmitted in Paul (6.13). There are marked similarities with the Arabic text, confirming (what the Arabic double quotation "Paul...Antyllus says" in Rāzī already suggests) that Paul's text is an excerpt from Antyllus. Paul's chapter can, therefore, be classified as an Antyllus fragment as well. The Arabic versions are excerpts of type 2 according to Weisser (1991).

## Fragment 1 on Trichiasis: Translations

| Translation from the Greek of Paul of Aegina 6.13 (ed. Heiberg 1921-1924 [CMG]) | Translation from the Arabic of Rāzī, Ḥāwī (I 87vII(14) Par. = 46rIIult. Ven. (book 2.6) = II.262.12 Haid.) | Translation from the Arabic of ʿAlī ibn ʿĪsā, II.10 (p. 102.10-104.2 ed. Khan, 1964, p. 81seq. Hirschberg & Lippert, 1904) |
|---|---|---|
| On *anabrochismós* We recommend the operation of *anabrochismós* in those who do not have lots of hairs on the eyelid that irritate the eye, but only one, two, or, at most, three that are close together. | **Paul.** And concerning the *anabrochismós* **Antyllus says:** | But as far as the *anabrochismós* and the sewing to the outside is concerned: |

| | | |
|---|---|---|
| Then we take an extremely thin needle and pull a woman's hair or a very simple linen thread through its needle eye, pulling the two ends simultaneously [through the needle eye] so that what is inserted forms a double loop. And we pass another thread of this type or a hair through the loop<br><br>and pull the needle through the edge of the eyelid, where the excess hairs appear.<br><br>**(Missing in Paul)** | Take an extremely thin needle and insert a woman's hair into its eye. And pull the two ends [of the hair] long to create a kind of loop. Then insert another hair into this eye [of the needle] because you need it.<br><br>Then position the patient on his neck and pull the eyelid towards you and pass the needle from the inside of the eyelid to its outside.<br><br>Then guide the needle and the hair so that no sort of little loop occurs at the inside of the eyelid, by the hair whose end is in the needle. | Take one of the needles of the cobblers, insert a woman's hair or a thin silk thread into its eye, pull the two ends [of the hair] long, so that a kind of loop is created. Then insert another hair into this needle eye because it is necessary.<br><br>Then make the patient lie down in front of you, lift his eyelid and pass the needle from the inner side of the eyelid to the outer one, at the edge of the eyelid, in the place where the excess hair has grown. |
| And we insert the hair or hairs into the loop using an ear probe and pull it [the loop] upwards. And when the eyelash is trapped, we pull up the loop. But if one or more slide out, then we pull the loop back downwards, using the thread that was additionally inserted, put the hair or hairs in again and pull them up. | Then take the hair that irritates, put it into that loop and push it away with a probe. Then lengthen the loop a little, while being tight, as far as it is possible. Then pull it with force so that the aforementioned hair comes to the outer eyelid. And the hair needs to go into the needle eye. | Then put it, be it one little hair or two, gradually into the loop and narrow the latter as much as possible; and now pull on quickly. |

| (Missing in Paul) | (Missing in Rāzī) | If the excess hair slips out when you pull on, the <second woman's> hair that is inside allows the loop to be pulled down <again>. Once the loop has come back down, insert the <sick> hair a second time <in it> and repeat your work until you have pulled the <sick> hair outwards. |
|---|---|---|
| But when it is a single hair that irritates the eye slightly, then we pull another of the eyelashes upwards, together with it, by coating it with rubber or some other glue-like substance and we connect them until the hairs stick together. Some, however, prefer cauterization to *anabrochismós*, whereby they evert the eyelid and pull out the irritating hair, be it one, two or three, with hair tweezers. They either set double-button probes, ear probes or a thin instrument of this type that has been made glowing in the fire on the spot from which they removed the hair or hairs. For this way no more hair grows out, because the skin becomes thicker. | And when it [the hair] has come out, apply wax to it several times so that it is not produced [again]. | When it is <just> one <single>, very fine hair, glue it to another of the <healthy> eyelashes so that it sticks to it, by gluing it with rubber or glue, until a connection [between both hairs] is created. Afterwards rub the probe on it repeatedly so that it does not become loose. |

| (Missing in Paul) | And you need the [second] hair that you [initially] put into the loop so that you can tighten the loop with it, if the hair does not come out gently, so that it is not cut and you have to repeat the *anabrochismós* procedure and so that a strong hair remains. But if you have to insert the needle a second time, do so in a different place. Because if you inserted it into that place for the second time, it [the hole] would expand and not hold the hair. | However, you need the <second woman's> hair, which you inserted into the loop in order to pull the loop back if the hair has not come out. Your procedure should be such that you handle the hair carefully so that it is not separated and you have to repeat the needle piercing. But if you have to insert the needle a second time, do so in a different place. Because if you inserted [the needle] into that place for the second time, it [the hole] would expand and not hold the hair. |

## Fragment 2 on Trichiasis: Commentary

This fragment is introduced by the author indication "Antyllus and Paul and what I [Rāzī] saw in the hospital." There is no parallel in Paul to this text. It seems to be an account of Rāzī's own clinical experience, based upon Antyllus. Since we lack any other fragment transmitting the pure Antyllus text, it is difficult to say what is based on Antyllus and what is Rāzī's own observation. At any rate, four possible forms of treatment for trichiasis are mentioned in this fragment: gluing, cauterizing, *anabrochismós,* and shortening of the eyelids. What follows is a comprehensive description of how to shorten the eyelids by removing a portion of skin from the outside.

**Fragment 2 on Trichiasis: Translation**

**Translation from the Arabic of Rāzī, Ḥāwī (I 87vI (1) Par. = 46rII (21) Ven. (book 2.6) = II.260.2 Haid.**

**Antyllus and Paul <and> what I saw in the hospital** about healing the excess hairs. **He says**: There are four kinds [of treatment]: gluing, cauterization, *anabrochismós,* and shortening of the eyelids. The best way to shorten the eyelids is as follows: If the eyelid has short eyelashes so that you cannot grasp them, insert a needle into the middle of the eyelid and insert a thread into it, with which you can grasp. Then grasp it, but with your index finger and thumb. Press the eyelid with a probe until it everts. Then incise its inside, in the place called the bowl. For it is similar to the cavity of a bowl. Incise it from one corner of the eye to the other one. Insert the threads into the eyelid, into the skin from above, in three places, one in the middle and two towards the corners of the eye. Then pull them [the threads] to you so that you can calculate the amount that is cut. When you see all the hairs have been removed and are coming out to the outside, and when you calculate the amount that is sufficient for you, then cut this amount so that no twisting [of the eyelid] is caused. Then cut this amount and suture it [the eyelid] in three places. The incision is only made on the outside of the skin of the eyelid. Apply the yellow powder on it by putting it on a compress, but to a certain measure. Place a compress moistened with vinegar and water on top to prevent swelling. In three days, he [the patient] will be cured. This is what I saw in the hospital.

**Fragment 3 on Trichiasis: Commentary**

This passage from Ṣalāḥ ad-Dīn excerpts a part of the aforementioned fragment 2 from Rāzī's Ḥāwī and also introduces this passage under the name "Antyllus and Paul." Then it continues with additional information—what to do if the surgeon has shortened the eyelid too much.

**Fragment 3 on Trichiasis: Translation**

> **Translation from the Arabic of Ṣalāḥ ad-Dīn,**
> **p. 183.18 (ed. al-Wafā'ī, 1987)**
>
> And its therapy [that of trichiasis] is like the therapy of the surplus hairs, as **Rāzī suggests in the second book of the Ḥāwī, taken from Antyllus and Paul.**
>
> **He says:** I saw in the hospital [the following] concerning the therapy of the <surplus> hairs: After having cut the eyelid, having sewn it, and having put the yellow powder and the compress on it, put a compress moistened with vinegar and water on the eyelid from upwards to prevent swelling. In three days, he [sc. the patient] will be cured. If the eyelid looks [too] short after you have shortened it excessively upwards, then use slackening substances such as water, fenugreek, pennyroyal, violet oil, and pure wax for external application. And when it [the eyelid] is flabby, rub [it] with strengthening astringent substances, such as acacia, green oak gall, myrtle, pomegranate flowers, and aloe. All this is mixed with the water of the myrtle and then applied. This is what can be said about the therapy of surplus and twisted hairs.

**Fragment 4 on Trichiasis: Commentary**

The last fragment on this topic is again preserved by Ṣalāḥ ad-Dīn. According to him, it is an excerpt from Rāzī's Ḥāwī and is said to have the author indication "from Antyllus and the 'Book of the Whole.'" However, this passage cannot be found in the edited Latin or Arabic text of the Ḥāwī (in terms of subject matter one would expect to find it in the fourth chapter of the second book of the Ḥāwī). Undoubtedly, Ṣalāḥ ad-Dīn's Ḥāwī copy was more complete than the printed editions available today. The content of the fragment is about an individual aspect of pharmaceutical therapy for trichiasis (excerpt of type 4 according to Weisser, 1991).

**Fragment 4 on Trichiasis: Translation**

> **Translation from the Arabic of Ṣalāḥ ad-Dīn,**
> **p. 301.14 (ed. al-Wafā'ī, 1987)**
>
> **The Sheikh (Ibn Sīnā) in the third book of the Canon and Rāzī in the Ḥāwī, from Antyllus and from the "Book of the Whole":** If a piercing in the conjunctiva occurs from blinking, then chew salt and cumin, do it [sc. the chewed mixture] in linen compresses, and wring it out into the eye. Then dip a piece of cotton[11] in egg white and rose oil, and place it on the eyelids. The leaves of the willow are also very useful as a dressing.

---

11 In Paul's Greek text, *érion* (= wool) is used, and in Celsus' cataract chapter (7.7.14), we find *lana* (= wool) in this context. In all Arabic authors, however, the Greek *érion* is translated by *quṭn* (= cotton). In Greek, *érion* can indeed mean cotton (= *érion apò xýlou*), but it may also have been the local practise of Arabic physicians to use cotton instead of wool, which made them translate *érion* as cotton.

**On Eyelid Inflammation/Loss of Eyelashes: Commentary**

Only one Arabic fragment about eyelid inflammation (*sulāq*) is transmitted (in Rāzī, Ḥāwī). In Greek, the loss of eyelashes due to eyelid inflammation is referred to by the name of *ptílōsis*. In Paul, a chapter on *ptílōsis* exists (Paul 3.22,17), which, however, has no parallel with the present fragment, which is an isolated, out-of-context statement of type 4 according to Weisser (1991). Interestingly, Antyllus is named an "Alexandrian" in this fragment (see the section on his biography).

**On Eyelid Inflammation/Loss of Eyelashes: Translation**

> **Translation from the Arabic of Rāzī, Ḥāwī (I 88vI (27)**
> **Par. = 46vIIu Ven. (book 2.6) = II.269.1 Haid.)**
>
> The treatment of the Alexandrian Antyllus for eyelid inflammation (*sulāq*) is amazingly beneficial. Take pine bark and Armenian stones and make a collyrium, because it conveys what makes the place grow where the eyelashes are.

**On Hydatid Cysts: Commentary**

Hydatids, as we know them in modern medical terminology, are echinococcal cysts that occur due to cystic echinococcosis, a parasitic disease. According to Antyllus' description, the ancient hydatids could well be echinococcal cysts, which can also occur on the eyelid, as described. The description of the symptomatology in Antyllus/Paul that the eyelids were edematous and flaccid and prevented the eyes from opening completely is entirely consistent with this. On the other hand, the characterization of hydatids as "fatty" seems strange, since echinococcal cysts tend to be whitish translucent and shiny. The remark in Greek that the hydatid lies "naturally" under the skin of the eyelid is also surprising. Since the ancients were not aware of the parasitic nature of this disease, it may have been assumed that a physiological structure might become hypertrophic and thereby pathological.

The chapter on hydatids preserved in Arabic bears the author indication "Antyllus and Paul." It is an almost complete rendering of Paul of Aegina's Greek text (the Arabic reproduction is, therefore, a type 1 quotation according to Weisser, 1991). There is no surplus text in Rāzī, compared to the Greek. The value of the Arabic fragments, therefore, lies in identifying the anonymous Paul chapter as an Antyllus excerpt. Considering the identical wording, 'Alī ibn 'Īsā apparently used the same Arabic translation of Antyllus, from which Rāzī excerpted.

**On Hydatid Cysts: Translations**

| Translation from the Greek of Paul of Aegina 6.14 (ed. Heiberg 1921-1924 [CMG]) | Translation from the Arabic of Rāzī, Ḥāwī (I 72rII Par. = 37rII Ven. (book 2.2) = II.136.ult.-137.16 Haid.) | Translation from the Arabic of ‘Alī ibn ‘Īsā, II,21 (p. 126 ed. Khan, 1964, p. 104seq. Hirschberg & Lippert, 1904) |
|---|---|---|
| On hydatid cysts The hydatid cyst is a sort of fatty structure that naturally lies under the skin of the eyelid. | The hydatid cyst. **Antyllus and Paul say:** This is a fatty mass that protrudes on the upper eyelid. And it prevents the eyelids from rising upwards. | The hydatid cyst ... it is a fatty and sticky mass ... and it protrudes on the outside of the upper eyelid. ... a thickening occurs on the outside of the upper eyelid, ... which prevents the eyelid from lifting completely. |
| However, in some people, and especially in children—since they have a moist constitution—it increases in size and becomes the cause of subsequent illnesses, as it presses on the eye and, for this reason, causes tear flow. The eyelids under the eyebrows [the upper eyelids] appear swollen and cannot be raised properly. | It occurs especially in boys, because of the moisture of their natures. And the upper eyelid becomes moist and flabby. | ... It occurs mostly in boys, because of the moisture of their natures; ... and the lids of their eyes are wet and flabby. |
| And when we press our fingers on them [the eyelids] and then spread our fingers, the space in between rises. | And if we press the place with the index and middle fingers and separate both [fingers], the middle between both of them protrudes. | And if you press the place with your index and middle fingers and then separate your fingers, what is between the two fingers will bulge out. |
| Early in the morning, they [the patients] suffer most from tear flow and they cannot look directly into the sun rays, but they water and are affected by constant inflammation of the eyes. | **He says:** And they suffer from catarrhs and have frequent tear flow. And they have frequent eye inflammations. | And they experience catarrhs and the constant flow of tears. This happens more often early in the morning. The patients cannot endure the shine of the sun for long, but tear flow quickly comes about ... and often they suffer from eye inflammation. |

| | | |
|---|---|---|
| We, therefore, position the patient in a suitable manner and press the eyelid with two fingers, namely, the index finger and the middle finger, slightly separated from each other, thereby creating a certain fixation of the hydatid cyst between the fingers.<br><br>We instruct the assistant, who stands behind and fixes the head, to pull up the eyelid slightly in the middle of the eyebrow. And we take a lancet and incise it [the eyelid] diagonally in the middle, making the incision not larger than for venesection, | The therapy: The patient should sit down, and an assistant should grasp his head and pull it backwards; and he should stretch the skin of the forehead near the eye so that the eyebrow rises. Then the physician should grasp the eyelid and its margins, in what is between the index and the middle finger. Then he should put a little pressure between these two fingers so that the moisture collects and it is pressed on what is between the fingers, while the assistant pulls the skin from the middle of the eyebrow. | The therapy: ... make the patient sit in front of you and place a man behind him to hold his head. ... and stretch the eyelid downwards; the assistant pulls the skin towards him until the cyst collects near the eyebrow; and instruct the one holding the head to pull the eyebrow up, until the cyst emerges. |
| but in terms of depth, we completely cut through the skin or even reach the hydatid cyst itself. We hereby carefully pay attention to the following: Many of those who penetrated too deeply have either severed the cornea or at least caused a muscle injury to the eyelid. And if the cyst becomes immediately visible, we extract it, otherwise we carefully cut again. | When we reach the hydatid cyst, or whatever is easier, we cut from the hydatid cyst with caution; for the ignorant person sometimes cuts the entire depth of the eyelid. This is what happens when it becomes visible to us. Otherwise we do it deep as well. And it is with the width until it [the hydatid cyst] appears. | (c) ... incise the area in which the cyst became visible with a lancet ... But this should be done gently. The ignorant person often cuts the eyelid too deeply. Hereby the eyelid cartilage is injured ...<br><br>(d) sometimes one of the eyelid muscles appears; that is bad ... |

| | | |
|---|---|---|
| But if it becomes visible, we grasp it with a soft compress with our fingers and extract it by moving it here and there and sometimes also circlewise. And after the removal, we soak a folded compress with vinegar water, apply it, and then bandage.<br>Some people also apply fine salt to the incision, using the button of the probe, in order to melt out what may be left of the hydatid cyst. | And when it appears, we wrap a cloth of linen on our fingers so that the hydatid cyst does not slip off our fingers. And we pull it right, left, and upwards until it comes out.<br><br>And if you think there is anything left of it, sprinkle salt on it so that the rest that is in it will be eaten up. And then put a wet compress with vinegar on it. | If it [the cyst] has now become visible to you, grasp it with a small piece of cloth, but be careful that it does not slip off your hand and stretch it ... to the right, to the left, and upwards, until it comes out entirely. ...<br><br>But if you have to assume that a remnant of it has remained inside, then fill the place with crushed salt so that it eats away and dissolves the rest. (d) |
| If the patients do not develop any inflammation after the removal, we treat them all over with ointment collyria, *Lycium*, *Glaucium*, or saffron. But if they have an inflammation, then we also treat them with cataplasms and other therapeutic aids. | And if it is the following day and you are safe from an inflammation, then treat with agglutinating medicines. And among them is *Lycium*, a collyrium, *Glaucium*, and saffron, until, God willing, he recovers. | ... treat them with acacia, *Lycium* and aroma, and aloe and *Glaucium* ointment ... along with a little saffron. |

## On Pterygium

Pterygium is still known by this name in modern medicine. It is a pathological wing-like membrane on the conjunctiva of the eye that may also extend to the cornea and thus impair vision. It was already known in ancient times that its growth usually originates from the nasal eye corner (see the initial remark by Paul, given in the text that follows).

## Fragment 1 on Pterygium: Commentary

Fragment 1 is introduced by the double author attribution "Antyllus and Paul" and represents an excerpt of type 2 according to Weisser (1991). The Greek text in Paul is more extensive and offers more information than the Arabic, except for one passage at the beginning that is missing in Greek, where the difference between two types of pterygia is described. Fragment 1 with its author indication in the form of a double quotation makes it possible to identify Paul's chapter 6.18 as an Antyllus excerpt.

**Fragment 1 on Pterygium: Translations**

| Translation from the Greek of Paul of Aegina 6.18 (ed. Heiberg 1921-1924 [CMG]) | Translation from the Arabic of Rāzī, Ḥāwī (I 72vI (16) Par. = 37vI Ven. (book 2.2) = II.138.1 Haid.) |
|---|---|
| On pterygia<br><br>This disease occurs when a sinewy membrane, usually starting from the large (ie, nasal) corner of the eye, gradually spreads inwards. It harms the eye in that it prevents its movement by contracting the eyeball and, if it progresses, completely covers the pupil. Since the delicate ones and those that shimmer white are quite easy to treat, we operate as follows: | **Antyllus and Paul and what I saw in a hospital. He says:** The pterygium. |
| **(Missing in Paul)** | The kind of it that is sticky gets scraped off when it sticks. And the (kind) of it that is not sticky requires a peeling. |
| We spread the eyelids, seize the pterygium with a slightly curved hook, and pull it upwards. | And its treatment is that you take a sharp hook (with) a small curve. Then the pterygium is pulled upwards with it. |
| Then we take a needle with a horse hair and a strong linen thread in its eye and which is slightly bent and pierce at the tip, below the middle of the pterygium, and tie the pterygium to the linen thread and then pull it upwards. But with the hair we, so to say, saw through the part near the pupil and peel it off to the end. But we cut out the rest of it, which is located at the large [nasal] corner of the eye, at its base with a scalpel for *anarrhaphé* [an operation by which the eyelid is sutured upward], leaving behind the natural piece of flesh at the corner of the eye [the lacrimal caruncle] so that no tear flow occurs when it is removed. Some people, however, as mentioned, pull it [the pterygium] upwards with the linen thread and peel the whole thing off with a pterygium scalpel, while taking care not to injure the cornea. | And a needle is inserted. Bend its eye a little and put a thread or a hair in it. Do this in one or two places, whichever seems better to us. And stretch it [the pterygium] <with the thread or hair [addition from the Latin version]> so that it is lifted (…). And if it [the pterygium] is not sticky, <remove it with the pannus> [correction according to the Latin version].<br><br>And if it is sticky, we peel it carefully off with a knife that is not sharp, but light. |

| After the operation, we sprinkle a little crushed salt on the area and bandage it with wool soaked in egg. After loosening [the bandage], we sprinkle it generously with salt water. But if an inflammation follows, we use the therapeutic means described for this purpose. | |
|---|---|

## Fragments 2 and 3 on Pterygium: Commentary

Fragments 2 and 3 have "Antyllus" alone as an author reference, without "Paul." Fragment 2 is an excerpt of type 3 according to Weisser (1991; an extensive passage condensed into a few sentences). Fragment 3 is of type 4 according to Weisser (1991; an isolated statement without further context). For both fragments, there are no parallels in Paul's chapter 6.18. Both fragments, therefore, appear to contain additional text excerpted directly from the Arabic Antyllus translation. Fragment 2 addresses the recurrence of the pterygium if it is not completely removed. Furthermore, the difference between pterygium and lacrimal caruncle is discussed as well as the postoperative treatment. 'Alī ibn 'Īsā excerpted the same text, probably from the Arabic Antyllus translation. Fragment 3 states that the pterygium sometimes adheres firmly to the "skin" of the eye (probably the conjunctiva, possibly also conjunctiva and cornea together) and that cutting the conjunctiva is dangerous.

| Translation from the Arabic of Rāzī, Ḥāwī (I 74vI Par. = 38vI Ven. (book 2.2) = II.150.14 Haid.) | Translation from the Arabic of 'Alī ibn 'Īsā, II.41 (p. 183seqq. ed. Khan, 1964, p. 152seq. Hirschberg & Lippert, 1904) |
|---|---|
| On the removal of the pterygium **Antyllus says:** If any remnant of it remains, it returns again; | ... leave nothing of <the substance of the> pterygium behind. Because if something is left behind, there will be a return. |
| and if it is removed without skill and if, along with it, the lacrimal caruncle, which is in the inner corner of the eye, is cut off, this results in frequent tear flow. | But be very careful not to take away the lacrimal caruncle, lest it results in tear flow. ... |
| And the difference between the lacrimal caruncle and the pterygium is that the pterygium is white and the lacrimal caruncle is dark and that the lacrimal caruncle is soft and the pterygium is hard. | (a) The difference between the <substance of the> pterygium and that of the lacrimal caruncle is that the pterygium appears white, hard, and sinewy, while the lacrimal caruncle, however, soft and red. (b) |

| And cut it off <with threads, like the vessels of the pannus [= trachoma pannus], as mentioned above, while flaying it with a quill. And when it is flayed, cut it … without the lacrimal caruncle> [addition from the Latin version]. | **Previously on p. 183 ed. Khan, 1964, p. 152 Hirschberg & Lippert, 1904:** … gently peel the <pterygium> off the conjunctiva. The quill is safer than any other <instrument> and causes no injury. … Once you have grasped it in the larger corner of the eye, cut it off with the scissors… |
|---|---|
| Then sprinkle salt and cumin into the eye and put egg white and rose oil into it. | Immediately following (a): (b) Then instill salt water with chewed cumin in the eye and bandage with egg yolk and rose oil… |
| Then, after a few days, apply red <collyria> on it [addition from the Latin version]. | When the third day is over, start the <after>treatment with… collyria and the like. |

**Fragment 3 on Pterygium: Translation**

| **Translation from the Arabic of Rāzī, Ḥāwī (I 72vI (9-16) Par. = 37rII.-2 Ven. (book 2.2) = II.137.17 Haid.)** | **Translation from the Greek of Aëtius of Amida 7.62 (ed. Olivieri, 1950, CMG VIII.2, p. 315.11-13)** |
|---|---|
| **Antyllus says:** And sometimes it (the pterygium) firmly adheres to the "skin" [ṣifāq, probably conjunctiva] of the eye. And then the "skin" [ṣifāq] comes out with it; and if it [the "skin"] is cut off, this is worrying. [Note: Probably because a part of the sclera is also removed.] | … so that the top layer of the cornea is not lifted. If it is removed, this will lead to very big inflammations. |

**Tumors and Fistulas of the Eye: *Aigilops* and *Anchilops*: Commentary**

Two sorts of periocular tumors are dealt with in the fragments of Antyllus' *cheir-ourgoúmena*: the so-called *aigilops* (lit. "goat's eye") and the *anchilops* (tumor "near the eye"). According to ancient ideas, both are similar and manifestations of the same disease, that is, a tumor on the nasal corner of the eye. According to Paul, the tumor is called *anchilops* as long as it is intact, whereas it is called *aigilops* as soon as it has broken open and started to spread to the surrounding area. Celsus (7.7.7. ed. Marx, 1915, CML I, p. 315) defines the disease as follows: "In the corner [of the eye] which is nearer to the nose a sort of small fistula opens up … through which slime flows constantly. The Greek call it *aigilops*. … Sometimes it goes beyond the bone and penetrates until the nose. Sometimes it has the property of a carcinoma, where the vessels are tense and curved …"

Adams (1844-47, vol. 2, pp. 284-286), Berendes (1914, p. 487), and Scheller and Frieboes (1967, p. 379) assume in their translations that it is a lacrimal sac fistula. The Arabs also seem to have understood it this way, translating *aigilops* as "fistula." However, with reference to Celsus, Magnus (1901, p. 399) rightly emphasizes that, according to modern pathology, *aigilops* is not a distinct disease, but rather a collective diagnosis: "By *aegilops* ophthalmologists understood ... not only diseases of the lacrimal sac, but in general all neoplasias in the area of the inner corner of the eye, such as warts, carcinomas, etc." The invasive variant, which also infiltrates bones and the nose, is probably a basal cell carcinoma, which occurs in areas of the body that are particularly exposed to solar (ultraviolet) radiation and spread locally (down to cartilage or bone) in a locally infiltrating or destructive manner. In the course of this, suppuration or fistula formation, as described for the *aigilops*, makes sense. *Anchilops* may be interpreted as a basal cell carcinoma in the early stages or as a fibroepithelioma.

In Arabic, the chapter on *aigilops* is entitled "Paul and Antyllus on the Fistula." However, a comparison with Paul's chapter 6.22 (On *Aigilops*) shows that the introductory sections, in which various forms of *aigilops* and the symptomatology are described, have no counterpart in Greek. Only in the section on surgical therapy do we see similarities of Weisser (1991) type 1. A special feature of the Arabic fragment is that, after the author reference "Paul and Antyllus," the sole reference "Paul" follows. The transition is not seamless, rather, starting with the author reference "Paul" an earlier stage of the description is taken up again.

If one compares the Arabic versions of Rāzī and 'Alī ibn 'Īsā, it becomes clear that 'Alī ibn 'Īsā excerpted from the same Arabic text as Rāzī, even if his text is significantly shortened compared to Rāzī.

## Aigilops and Anchilops: Translations

| Translation from the Greek of Paul 6.22 (ed. Heiberg 1921-1924 [CMG]) | Translation from the Arabic of Rāzī, Ḥāwī (I 85vII below Par. = 45rII Ven. (book 2.5) = II.249.5 Haid.) | Translation from the Arabic of 'Alī ibn 'Īsā, II.34 (pp. 153.9-155.2 ed. Khan, 1964, p. 125 Hirschberg & Lippert, 1904) |
|---|---|---|
| On the *aigilops*<br><br>The aigilops is an abscess-like tumor located between the large (ie, nasal) corner of the eye and the nose. The disease is difficult to treat because of the delicacy of the structures and the fear of a simultaneous affection [sympathy] of the eye. | Paul and Antyllus on the "fistula."<br>**Antyllus says:** A tumor occurs from the larger corner of the eye. And sometimes it protrudes outwards so that you can see its noticeable swelling. And sometimes it is turned inwards so that its swelling does not show at all. | But you must know that there is a type of lacrimal tumor that does not protrude outwards at all and in which no abscess appears at all; and another type that protrudes outwards and in which you can clearly see the swelling. |

| | | |
|---|---|---|
| **(Greek equivalent missing)** | And in the kind that is visible, pus flows from it and the flesh does not putrefy. And sometimes [the tumor] spreads to the nose and there is a species of it that spreads to the eye. And sometimes it spreads to both sides, to the inside and to the outside. | |
| **(Greek equivalent missing)** | And there are some that are very concave and some that do not extend deeply. <And the deep [tumor] causes the bone to rot.> [added from the Latin version]. And the one that is not great in depth does not cause the bone to rot. And sometimes the entire bone of the nose rots. | The one that does not penetrate deeply does not destroy the bone either. But the one that goes deeply destroys the bone, and sometimes even destroys the entire nasal bone. |
| **(Greek equivalent missing)** | And in the [kind] of it that protrudes outwards, healing is easy, especially if there is an opening in it from which there is secretion. And regarding the one that is turned towards the eye: Its symptom is the pain that suddenly appears in the eye at any moment without cause and the flowing of tears from the corner of the eye. It is inevitable that pus will flow from the corners of the eyes when you press on them. | The one that protrudes outwards is easier to treat, |

| | | |
|---|---|---|
| If the abscess is broken up on the surface, we excise everything that protrudes down to the bone. And if the abscess extends towards the jaw, then we open it completely and scrape the bone that is still intact. | The treatment: If the tumor is not deep and not chronic, the bone is not corrupted and you can excise it [the tumor]. And if it does not penetrate to the bone, then completely remove from the bone what is corrupted and make the rest heal. | especially if it has not yet become chronic. Then you have to incise it. If it does not reach the bone, then take away all the affected flesh and rasp the bone and apply ointment to scar the rest. |
| We burn the putrefied bone with a button cautery, placing a sponge soaked in cold water on the eye. Some, however, have used a drill after cutting out the fleshy parts, draining the fluid or pus into the nose. But we contented ourselves with burning alone, cauterizing with *aigilops* cauteries until a bone chip detaches. | And in case it reaches the bone, cauterize it until you get to the bone; and cauterize the bone until its cortex detaches from it. And destroy the rotten flesh. And if you do not want to cauterize it, then [use] the sharp medicines | But when it has reached the bone... then burn with small cauteries ... Cauterize until the corroded cortex falls off the bone...If you choose a sharp medicine instead of burning, then do so. ... |
| **(see once more before)** | **Paul says:** When the tumor is turned outwards, then cut into it and dry the flesh until you get to the bone. And if the bone is not affected, scrape it off; and if it is affected, then cauterize it after applying a sponge with ice water on the eye. And some people make an opening, when the flesh begins to putrefy, to let the pus flow into the nose. We content ourselves with only cauterizing it. | |
| And after cauterization, we use a mixture of lentils and honey, the medicine of pomegranate peel, and the other drying remedies. | | |

| | | |
|---|---|---|
| But if the *aigilops* creeps to the corner of the eye and also to the surface, but not completely, we use a pterygium or vein lancet to detach the tissue in the middle of the corner of the eye towards the abscess, bring the fleshy parts up from the depth and then dry them a little [with medicaments]. Finely powdered glass[12] applied to them dries them miraculously and aloe with incense in the same way. | **He says:** And if the tumor of the eye tends to the corner of the eye and is not deep, then we cut from the tumor to the corner of the eye; and take away what is found of corrupted flesh. And dry it with medicines. And a substance that amazingly causes this drying is glass when you grind it into dust and sprinkle it on the [affected] spot. And also aloe, if you crush it with the bark of incense. | |

## On *Anchilops*: Commentary

In the chapter on *anchilops* Antyllus (as quoted by Rāzī) points out that it is a type of lacrimal tumor "that does not spread to the eye or to the nose," that is, which is not locally invasive or infiltrating. For the difference between *aigilops* and *anchilops*, see the previous section.

Regarding the symptoms, it is stated that no pus evacuates from the nose or eyes when pressure on the tumor is made. However, the patients do have discomfort, feel pain, and have ongoing inflammation or tear flow from the eyes.

On comparing it with Rāzī, it is apparent that the version of 'Alī ibn 'Īsā is once again based on the same original source and that it is more detailed. In addition to the therapy through incision mentioned by Rāzī, 'Alī ibn 'Īsā also mentions purely pharmaceutical treatment and therapy through cauterization.

---

12 *Hýalos chnoódēs.* The authors of the Greek-English dictionary by Liddell-Scott-Jones do not give an exact meaning for this term. With reference to this very passage, they write: "Paul. Aeg. 6.22, is an absorbent of some kind." Hýalos is used not only for glass but also for alabaster and rock salt; it could, therefore, be a sort of powdered salt or gypsum

**On Anchilops: Translations.**

| Translation from the Arabic of Rāzī, Ḥāwī (I 87rI Par. = 46rI Ven. (book 2.5) = II.257.10 Haid.) | Translation from the Arabic of ʿAlī ibn ʿĪsā, II,34 (pp. 151.6-152.3 ed. Khan, 1964, p. 123 Hirschberg & Lippert, 1904) |
|---|---|
| **Antyllus says:** There is a type of lacrimal tumor [*ġarab*] that does not spread to the eye or to the nose. And it is just an outgrowth from the corners of your eye. | And sometimes there is a kind of lacrimal tumor [*ġarab*] that does not spread at all: |
| And when you squeeze it, no pus comes out, either from the corners of the eyes or from the nose. And the patient feels pain from it and [the eye] begins to be inflamed all the time without reason. | When you squeeze it, no pus comes out, either from the corner of the eye or from the nose. But the patient feels pain, both of his eyes are constantly suffering from inflammation, without any visible cause. The <affected> place swells, including the eyelids, and becomes small again and stops <swelling> completely ... |
| And tears seep out. And about this, you should know that the tumor does not spread to the eye. | |
| Cut it and treat it [with medicaments] | The treatment is done in three ways: first by medicaments ... secondly by burning, and thirdly by piercing. |

# Section 3: Antyllus on the Cataract

A cataract[13] is an opacity of the lens of the eye, caused by a multitude of reasons, including, as we know today, metabolic diseases, diseases of the skin and the eyes, trauma, or structural changes of the lens due to aging. It was only Pierre Brisseau in 1706 who identified a lenticular opacity as the cause of cataract. Previously, it had been thought (since antiquity in fact) that a cataract was due to a fluid gathering between the iris and the lens and coagulating there—hence the ancient Greek term *hypóchyma* (lit. "dispersion [of fluid] underneath") for cataract.[14] Surgical therapy for cataracts by couching was known at least since the 3rd century BC, as is clear from a reference to the philosopher Chrysippus (281/77-208/4) in Simplicius' commentary on Aristotle's *Categories*[15]: "Chrysippus asked whether people with cataract should be called blind, since they can see again after a couching [of the cataract]." Couching of the cataract was practiced from antiquity until the first half of the 20th century[16]—in some Third World countries, it is still performed today. The operation consists in piercing a cataract needle through the sclera and using it to depress the opaque lens. According to the ancient understanding of the disease, physicians in antiquity and the Middle Ages did not understand that they were couching the lens itself. Rather, they thought that they were couching the alleged opaque substance in front of it. Descriptions of the cataract operation are transmitted in Celsus (7.7.13-7.14) (1st century BC), the veterinary manual *Mulomedicina Chironis*[17] (71-76) (around 400 AD) as well as in Paul of Aegina (6.21) (7th century AD). All three sources are compilations rather than original texts and, therefore, draw their material from older sources.

Apart from that, 11 fragments on cataract surgery by Antyllus (approximately 2nd century AD) have been transmitted in Arabic translation. Antyllus' cataract fragments are edited here in English translation for the first time. They are, as well, excerpts, (more or less direct) reflections, or summaries of a chapter on cataract surgery from book 1 of Antyllus' lost surgical manual *cheirourgoúmena*.

**Fragments from Antyllus' Chapter on Cataracts: Commentary**

Eleven fragments of Antyllus' chapter on the cataract and its surgical treatment have come down to us, as excerpts in Arabic medical treatises: four in Rāzī's Ḥāwī (fragments 1-3 and 8), two in ʿAlī ibn ʿĪsā (fragments 4 and 6), four in Ṣalāḥ ad-Dīn (fragments 5, 7, and 9), and two in Ḥalīfa (fragments 10 and 11).

---

13  For the history of this technical term, see Fischer (2000).

14  See Meyerhof (1933), p. 73.

15  See Simplicius, *In Arist. categ. comm.* (ed. Kalbfleisch [1907]), p. 401, ln. 7seqq, and Meyerhof (1933), p. 72.

16  See Meyerhof (1932), p. 118.

17  See Fischer (2006), pp. 203-224 (pp. 211-216: 2. Die Staroperation).

Of all Antyllus fragments, those on the cataract have received the greatest attention from medical historians so far. This is particularly due to the 19th-century ophthalmologist and medical historian Julius Hirschberg who published widely on the history of ophthalmology (Hirschberg, 1904, 1906, 1918). Apart from fragment 2, the first part of fragment 1 and fragment 6, which escaped the attention of previous scholars, all other fragments have already been (partially) translated, commented on, or paraphrased, sometimes by several authors.[18] However, a complete English translation, based on the Arabic original, as is given here, was not available so far.

**Fragment 1 on Cataract: Translations**

| Translation from the Greek of Paul of Aegina 6.21 (ed. Heiberg 1921-1924 [CMG]) | Translation from the Arabic of Rāzī, Ḥāwī (I 78vI Par. = 41rI Ven. (book 2.3) = II.181.5 Haid.) |
|---|---|
|  | On the cataract, by Antyllus and Paul<br><br>Paul says: … |
| **(No exact Greek equivalent)** Cf. Paul (1): The plaster- and hail-like [color], however, occurs in the excessively solidified ones. (2.) | **Antyllus says:** The cataract that is colored like gypsum and the very black one are both bad (and) not suitable for being couched. |
| [ibid., further above]: … In the solidified [cataracts], however, no change occurs through lateral pressure, neither in width nor in shape. | **He says:** And couching of the congealed cataract, which does not fluctuate upon compression and does not deviate from its form, is useless. Because the intensely congealed cataract does not remain [in its position] when it has been removed from the eye. However, it does not immediately return and disappear, because it is very smooth and has no moisture in it. |

---

18 In the following, it is indicated by what scholars the single Antyllus fragments on the cataract have been translated or commented upon so far. The abbreviation [ar.] means that the scholar worked with the Arabic text, [lat.] means that he used the Latin version. Since Hirschberg published the same material in a number of publications, partly identically, partly with minor changes and additions, such a general view seems justified. Fragment 1 (second half): Meyerhof (1933) p. 75seq. [ar.]; fragment 3: Hirschberg (1906) p. 98 [ar.], Hirschberg (1918) p. 115 [ar.], Meyerhof (1932) pp. 116-118 [ar.], Meyerhof (1933) p. 74seq. [ar.]; fragment 4: Hirschberg/Lippert (1904) pp. 213-236 [ar.]; fragment 5: Hirschberg/Lippert/Mittwoch (1905) pp. 252-254 [ar.]; fragment 7: Hirschberg/Lippert/Mittwoch (1905) p. 241 [ar.]; fragment 8: Pansier (1903), p. 77 [lat.], Hirschberg (1904) p. 226 [lat.], Hirschberg (1906) p. 99 [ar.], Hirschberg (1918) p. 116 [ar.], Meyerhof (1932) p. 118 [ar.], Meyerhof (1933) p. 77 [ar.]; fragment 9: Pansier (1903) p. 80 [ar.], Hirschberg (1904) p. 227 [ar.], Hirschberg/Lippert/Mittwoch (1905) p. 261seq. [ar.], Hirschberg (1905) pp. 230, 231 [ar.], Hirschberg (1906) p. 99 [ar.]; fragment 10: Hirschberg (1904) p. 227 [ar.], Hirschberg (1905) p. 232 [ar.]; fragment 1q: Hirschberg (1904) p. 227 [ar.], Hirschberg (1905) p. 232 [ar.].

| | |
|---|---|
| **(No Greek equivalent)** | **He says:** And some kind of cataract never congeals, whereas [another kind] of it congeals after many years. And that [kind] of it should be couched, which is evenly congealed. The excessively diluted one should not be couched. And a sign of the diluted cataract is that it is dispersed with pressure and squeezing. And a sign of the hardened one is that it does not move at all. And a sign of the moderately hardened one is that it expands after it occurred. Then it returns to its shape. |
| Cf. Paul (1): The plaster- and hail-like [color], however, occurs in the excessively solidified ones. (2.) [Before:] what appears steel like, dark, and lead-like is the color of the moderately solidified cataracts. | **He says:** And the cataract that is colored like a hailstone and the intensely white one should not be couched because they are intensely congealed. And the lead-colored cataract should be couched because [the color] indicates that it [has] a moderate degree of condensation. |
| (2.) … We make the patient sit facing the light, but not in direct sunlight;<br><br>we carefully bandage the healthy eye, spread the lids of the other one,<br><br>keep distance from the so-called iris to the small corner of the eye, approximately according to the length of the button of the probe; | The treatment<br>**He says:** The patient should sit in the shade opposite the sun because the cataract can be seen clearly in that place. For in the sun or in much light, it [the cataract] is not visible. And his healthy eye shall be bandaged, lest he [the patient] escapes from what he sees; and instruct the patient to look to the "large" angle of his eye, towards his nose, and not to the "small" angle. Then keep distance from the black of the eye, according to the length of the tip of the probe.<br>**By me [Rāzī]:** This is done so that the cataract needle, when going in[to the eye], reaches only the opening of the uvea. |

| | |
|---|---|
| then we press the spot where we want to perform the couching with the button of the cataract needle<br><br>(using the right hand for the left eye and the left one for the right, [missing in Arabic])<br><br><br><br>and we turn the tip of the cataract needle, which is rounded at the end, forward by applying constant pressure on it [the cataract needle], through the spot previously indented, until it [the cataract needle] goes into the void [until a sudden decrease of resistance is felt].<br>A measure for penetrating into the depth be as much as the distance between the pupil and the iris. | **He says:** And mark that place with the [ie, blunt] tail of the cataract needle, by pressing on it until there is a pit in it [the sclera]. And this is done for two reasons: firstly, so that the patient gets accustomed to perseverance and tests it, and secondly, so that a place is created for the sharp tip [of the probe] in which it is fixed and from which it does not slide away, if we push it [the needle] with momentum. Afterwards, the sharp tip [ie, of the needle] is placed on that spot, then press forcefully until you feel the star needle go into the void [*áchri kenembatéseōs*,[19] ie, until a sudden decrease in resistance is felt].<br><br><br><br>And it is necessary that the depth of the insertion of the cataract needle equals the measure of the distance from the uvea [*recte*: iris] to the end of the pupil. |
| Afterwards, we direct the cataract needle to the top of the cataract—since you can see the bronze [sc. the needle] clearly because of the transparency of the cornea—<br><br>and bring with its [the needle's] help the cataract to the underlying parts. Immediately after it [the cataract] has been couched, we stay a little [with the needle] and do not move it. If the cataract rises again, we couch it downwards once more. | **He says:** After that, direct the cataract needle above the cataract. The bronze is visible due to the clarity of the cornea. Afterwards, direct it [the cataract needle] downwards, into the posterior part of the cornea membrane, where the cataract is situated, push it [the cataract] downwards and press the cataract needle firmly on it [= the cataract], for a short time. Then lift it [= the needle] up. If the cataract rises [again], depress it once again, until it does not rise any more. |
| Having couched the cataract, we carefully pull out the cataract needle while turning it. | Then gradually pull out the cataract needle while turning it. |

---

19 The Greek term *kenembátēsis* (lit. "entering the void") is used in a figurative sense in medical authors. The Greek-English Lexikon by Liddle/Scott/Jones translates it as "piercing of a cavity." What is meant by this term, however, is a sudden decrease in resistance that is felt when puncturing a cavity or cyst. The Arabic translation "until you feel the star needle go into the void" is a literal translation of the term *kenembátēsis*.

| | |
|---|---|
| Afterwards, we dissolve a little bit of Cappadocian salt in water and instill it [the solution] into the eye. And from outside we apply wool that has been soaked in egg yolk and rose oil and then we bandage; we bandage the healthy eye as well so that [the operated one] is not moved. And we make the patient lie in a subterranean room and instruct him not to move at all, administering him a light diet and keeping him bandaged up to the seventh day if nothing contradicts.<br><br>Then we loosen the bandage and test his eyesight by showing him visible objects. We advise against doing this during or immediately after surgery because the cataract may easily rise again as a result of the intense visual strain. In case any inflammation forces us to do so, we also remove the bandage before the seventh day and fight it [the inflammation]. | Afterwards, instill some salt and water into the eye, rinse the eye with it, and put a piece of cotton with egg yolk and rose oil on it.<br><br>Bandage it and bandage the healthy eye together with it so that it does not move the other one with its movement. And put the patient in a dark room. He should avoid sneezing, speaking, and violent movements. And his food should be light until the seventh [day]. And the bandage should remain in its place until that day, unless some impediment such as pain or a warm swelling prevents it. Then it [the bandage] is removed and one should test whether he [the patient] sees. And do not test whether he can see right away after couching the cataract, because that causes the cataract to rise quickly, because the patient looks through the eye with effort. And if some inconvenience occurs to him, unbandage the eye before the seventh [day]. And remedy what has happened. |
| **(No Greek equivalent)** | **Antyllus says:** When the cataract needle penetrates, the sharp tip [of the needle] should be inclined to the "small" [eye] angle, because this way it leaves the remaining membranes intact. Then turn it [the cataract needle] gradually until you get it over the cataract. After that, couch it [the cataract] downwards. |

|  | **He says:** However, if the cataract is cloudy and difficult to couch, if it stays couched at first and [then] returns back, then disperse it with the cataract needle to all sides. It might be that it is [this way] completely cured. And push it to the "small" or to the "big" eye angle or upwards. And observe at which place it can be reached better [with the needle] and gets attached. Then push it [the needle]. And it often gets attached at the top. So the patient is healthy and it [the cataract] does not revert.<br>**He says:** You should know that sometimes the cataract needle goes too far [so that] blood leaks out and clots in the puncture site of the eye. And this causes a condition that does not heal at all. |
|---|---|
| Cf. Paul (2.): And from outside we apply wool that has been soaked in egg yolk and rose oil and then we bandage; we bandage the healthy eye as well so that [the operated one] is not moved.<br><br>**(No Greek equivalent)**<br><br><br>… keeping him bandaged up to the seventh day if nothing contradicts. | **He says:** And after couching the cataract, dress both eyes simultaneously. Apply to both [eyes] rose oil and egg. And remove it [the dressing] only after three days have elapsed, provided that no pain or swelling causes you to do so [earlier]. And when you remove them [the dressings], heat them a little using warm poultices on them, with boiled rose water or willow leaves. Do this until the seventh day and until pain ceases completely; then remove it [the dressing]. And if the cataract returns at some time during these days, insert the cataract needle again into this puncture site, into the same puncture channel, not into another one, because that puncture site is not completely scarred, because it is in the "cartilage." |

## Fragment 1 on Cataract: Commentary

Fragment 1 is introduced by the heading "Antyllus and Paul on the cataract." What follows is a section introduced by "Paul says," followed by two passages with the introductory remark "Antyllus says." The introductory excerpt from Paulus (omitted here) corresponds almost completely to the first section of Paul's chapter 6.21 (excerpt of Weisser [1991] type 1).

The following section, solely assigned to Antyllus, deals with different types of cataracts, their characteristics, and suitability for couching. There are no direct Greek equivalents or corresponding portions for this passage in Paul, except for some vague echoes in the first section of his cataract chapter. The subsequent part on therapy, however, still quoted under the name of Antyllus, is an almost complete rendition of the second and last sections of Paul's chapter 6.21. The subsequent last section of fragment 1, again introduced with "Antyllus says," contains certain technical details about couching the cataract and handling the cataract needle, terminating with a section on postoperative care. A Greek equivalent in Paul is missing, once again. What follows—still under Antyllus' name—is the description of the actual operation. It almost completely reproduces the second section of Paul's cataract chapter 6.21, up to the end. This is followed by a further section on the operation (again introduced with "Antyllus says: ..."), which begins at an earlier stage of the operation (the penetration of the cataract needle into the eye) and continues again until the description of postoperative aftercare. This section shows almost no parallels with Paul and describes details of the treatment that are not known from any Greek source.

All in all, it becomes clear that Paul's chapter 6.21 is obviously an excerpt from Antyllus' cataract chapter,[20] whereas Antyllus' descriptions were more extensive and Paul only excerpted a part of them.

---

20  This has already been pointed out by Hirschberg/Lippert p. 299, fn. 4.

**Fragment 2 on Cataract: Translations**

| Translation from the Greek of Paul of Aegina 6.21 (ed. Heiberg 1921-1924 [CMG]) | Translation from the Arabic of Rāzī, Ḥāwī (I 79rII,-2 Par. = 41vI Ven. (book 2.3) = II.200.3 Haid.) |
|---|---|
| (1.) … it [the cataract] occurs primarily because of a cooling or weakness of the optic *pneuma* … | **Antyllus says:** The cataract occurs in the eye. It is caused by coldness of the [body's] mixture, coldness of the air [= optic *pneuma*], and humidity of the eye. And the kind of [cataract] can be couched, which is moderately condensed. The condensed one, however, and the one which is too smoothly dispersed are not couched. |
| We close the eye with the cataract, press the eyelid with the thumb against the eye, and move it [sc. the eyelid] here and there, while pressing it. Then we open it, observe it with our eye, and have a look at the cataract: In the [cataracts] that have not yet solidified, a kind of effusion is produced additionally, as a result of the pressing with the finger; and at the beginning, it [the cataract] appears wider, then it returns to its original shape and size. In the solidified [cataracts], however, no change occur through lateral pressure, neither in width nor in shape. … | And the following kind of cataract is condensed: When you press your thumb on the eyelid, move it [the lid], lift the eyelid, and notice that it [the cataract] does not disperse but does return and stay in its condition and does not move. |
| Because what appears steel-like, dark, and lead-like is the color of the moderately solidified ones. And they are suitable for couching. The plaster- and hail-like [colors], however, occur in the excessively solidified ones. (2.) | And the cataract whose color is the color of iron and lead is moderately condensed and should be couched. And the one whose color is like gypsum or ice is intensely condensed and should not be couched. |
| | **By me [sc. Rāzī]:** Have a look at this [topic] in the *Book of the Collection*. The patient who has a cataract in his eye must not vomit [must not be administered vomitives], because it [the vomiting] brings to it [the eye] a residual substance. |

**Fragment 2 on Cataract: Commentary**

Fragment 2, again marked as an Antyllus excerpt ("Antyllus says: ..."), represents a slightly shortened version of the first section of Paul's chapter 6.21 (Weisser [1991] type 2) and has no surplus passages compared to Paul's Greek text.

**Fragment 3 on Cataract: Translations**

| Translation from the Greek of Paul of Aegina 6.21 (ed. Heiberg 1921-1924 [CMG]) | Translation from the Arabic of Rāzī, Ḥāwī (I 79vI Par. = 41vI Ven. (book 2.3) = II.200.11 Haid.) |
|---|---|
| (2.) ... We make the patient sit facing the light, but not in direct sunlight;<br><br>**(No Greek equivalent)** | **Antyllus on couching the cataract**<br>**He says:** The patient should sit in the shade and in a place where his face is opposite the solar disc.<br>Then hold his head and instruct him to turn his pupil to the "greater" [nasal] angle of the eye, looking towards you, similar to looking sideways to the "smaller" [temporal] angle of the eye. |
| we ... keep distance from the so-called iris to the small corner of the eye, corresponding approximately to the length of the button of the probe;<br><br>then we press the spot where we want to perform the couching with the button of the cataract needle ... | **He says:** And keep the distance from the black of the eye according to the measure of the tip of the cataract needle so that, when the tip is completely in the eye, it reaches the pupil. Then take a probe with a broad head and make an impression at the place where you want to insert the cataract needle so that a pit is made there and the pin of the cataract needle does not slip away when you press on it. |
| (*) A measure for penetrating into the depth be as much as the distance between the pupil and the iris. (*)<br><br><br>**(No Greek equivalent)** | And the size of the head of the cataract needle should correspond to the distance to the pupil or exceed it by the size of a barley grain and should not be longer than it. For if it (sc. the head of the cataract needle) is longer, then attach something on it [= as a break stop]. And it is best if those buttons [= break stops] are made from brass. Mount them [on the cataract needle] and remove them, if you want. |

| | |
|---|---|
| and we turn the tip of the cataract needle, which is rounded at the end, forward by applying constant pressure on it [the cataract needle], through the spot previously indented, until it [the cataract needle] goes into the void (ie, until a sudden decrease in resistance is felt). (*) [passage (*)-(*) following]<br><br>**(No Greek equivalent)**<br><br>Afterwards, we bring the cataract needle to the top of the cataract … and bring with its [the needle's] help the cataract to the underlying parts. Immediately after it [the cataract] has been couched, we stay a little [with the needle] and do not move it. If the cataract rises again, we couch it downwards once more. | Then press on the cataract needle until the conjunctiva and cornea are pierced. For the uvea is pushed back by it [the cataract needle], but it is not pierced because it has a sticky surface. And the tip of the cataract needle should not be sharp. And when the cataract needle enters, put your mouth [some manuscripts: a piece of cotton] on the eye and suck it [some manuscripts: close it] until the pupil is even. And leave the cataract needle in its place. Then open it [the eye] and have a look where its tip [the tip of the needle] is pointing. If it has not reached the location of the cataract yet, push it [the needle] a little. And when it [the needle] has passed it [the cataract], pull it back a little until it is on the same level as the cataract. Having done this, gradually lift the lower part of the cataract needle. Then push on its head. Do not stop doing this with the tail of the cataract needle, as long as it is necessary. Your aim should be to push the cataract down. If it [the cataract] is difficult [in that] it returns after you have couched it, then disperse it sideways, where it is easy for you to do so, until he [the patient] can suddenly see. |
| Having couched the cataract, we carefully pull out the cataract needle while turning it.<br>… And from outside we apply wool that has been soaked in egg yolk and rose oil and then we bandage; | And when you have finished, <pull the cataract needle out> and apply egg white and rose oil to the eye for three days. And he [the patient] should always lie on his back. After that, anoint it [the eye] with the white collyrium, because the eye is irritated in any case. |
| we bandage the healthy eye as well so that [the operated one] is not moved. | And when you perform the couching of the cataract, bandage the eye that is not going to be operated. And also when [the patient] is sleeping on his back, the other eye should be bandaged. |

| | |
|---|---|
| And we make the patient lie in a subterranean room and instruct him not to move at all, … keeping him bandaged up to the seventh day if nothing contradicts. … In case that any inflammation forces us to do so, we also remove the bandage before the seventh day and fight it [the inflammation].<br><br>**(No Greek equivalent)** | And let him [the patient] sleep in a dark room and observe him closely so that you recognize his condition. And make sure that he does not have to sneeze, that he does not speak or cough, and that he does not untie it [the bandage] until the third day, unless something happens that makes it necessary.<br>And if you need to reinsert the cataract needle into it [the eye], do it through the same hole in his eye, because it does not scar quickly. |

## Fragment 3 on Cataract: Commentary

Fragment 3 is headed "Antyllus on couching the cataract" in Arabic and gives the impression of an excerpt of Weisser (1991) type 1. Essentially, it corresponds to the second section of Paul's chapter 6.21. Fragment 3 is, however, more detailed than Paul's corresponding text, and some of its passages lack a Greek equivalent.

## Fragment 4 on Cataract: Translations

| Translation from the Greek of Paul of Aegina 6.21 (ed. Heiberg 1921-1924 [CMG]) | Translation from the Arabic of 'Alī ibn 'Īsā II.73-74 (p. 254.13 ed. Khan, 1964) |
|---|---|
| On cataracts<br>(1.) A cataracts is a collection of inert fluid on the cornea at the pupil, which prevents vision or clear vision.<br><br><br>But it arises primarily because of a cooling or weakness of the optic pneuma, and for this reason, it is more likely to occur in old people and in those who suffer from a chronic illness. It also occurs due to violent vomiting, as a result of a blow and of several other causes. … | Sometimes, a disease occurs between the layer of the uvea and the cornea membrane, which is called "cataract." And it consists in a congealed fluid at the front of the pupil... (256.7). This fluid comes about for several reasons: It arises as a result of violent vomiting or as a result of a blow or an impact on the head or the eye. And often it occurs because of severe cold. It also occurs because of a weakness of the optic pneuma. Therefore, it frequently occurs in elderly people, because the congenital heat and pneuma are weakened in them. And it [the disease] occurs in those suffering from a chronic illness. It occurs because of constant ingestion of moist and thick foodstuffs. It also occurs as a result of chronic headaches and also because of the coldness of the body mixture. |

| | And it occurs because of many other causes. And most often, it occurs in dark eyes because their moisture is greater. .. |
| --- | --- |
| All cataract patients see either excessive or little brightness. We hereby distinguish the cataract from the amaurosis and *glaucoma*, since patients with amaurosis and *glaucoma* do not see any brightness at all. … | **(No Arabic equivalent)** |
| We close the eye with the cataract, press the eyelid with the thumb against the eye, and move it [the eyelid] here and there, while pressing it. Then we open it, observe it with our eye, and have a look at the cataract:<br><br>In the [cataracts] that have not yet solidified, a kind of effusion is produced additionally, as a result of the pressing with the finger; and at the beginning, it [the cataract] appears wider, then it returns to its original shape and size. In the solidified [cataracts], however, no change occurs through lateral pressure, either in width or in shape.<br><br>But since this is a common feature of the moderately solidified and excessively solidified [cataracts], we distinguish them by their color. Because what appears steel-like, dark and lead-like is the color of the moderately solidified ones. And they are suitable for couching. The plaster-like and hail-like [color], however, occurs in the excessively solidified ones. | (260.9) The sign that [sc. the cataract] is "grown in" [solidified]: Let the patient stand in front of you in the sun, close the eye with the cataract, press the patient's eyelid with [your] thumb, and move it [the cataract] sidewards and back [lit.: to this side and to that side]. Then open the eye and examine the condition of the cataract. And if it was not yet "grown in" or condensed, the following happens: As soon as you press it with your fingers, it will dilate and become wider than it was before; thereafter, it returns to its original shape. But when it has become condensed and consolidated, it shows no change at all when being compressed, concerning both its breadth and its shape.<br><br>And this is a common sign of the [cataract] that has become condensed and uniformly thick, as well as of [the cataract] that has become excessively condensed, that no change occurs [upon compression]. Among the [signs] that indicate that it is good as for its substance and uniform as for its thickness is its color, which must be like that of steel or lead. However, the color of the cataract that is already completely solidified is similar to that of gypsum or that of a hailstone |

| | |
|---|---|
| (2.) ... We make the patient sit facing the light, but not in direct sunlight; | ... (270.7). Make the patient sit in the shade, facing the light, opposite the sun, after you had previously evacuated him with purgatives, by venesection of the vein of the elbow and by purgation of the head and the body, as much as you can. Let the day be one with northern wind and not with southern one,[21] and let it be a sunny day. ... Have the patient sit on a soft pillow and bring his knees to his chest, and tie his hands together on his thighs. Sit on a chair so that you are positioned higher than him, of medium height. |
| we carefully bandage the unaffected eye,<br><br><br><br><br><br><br><br>spread the lids of the other one, | And bandage his healthy eye very tightly with a compress of moderate thickness. Because there are two benefits: The first is that the eye does not move at the time of healing by stimulating its movement through the movement of the other one. The other benefit is if your treatment is successful and you let the patient whose cataract has been couched see something, you are not told that he [the patient] sees with his healthy [eye]. And instruct a person [an assistant] to stand behind him and to hold his head. Then he [the assistant] should elevate the upper lid of his [the patient's] eye until it separates from the lower lid and he should thus make the whole eye visible to you.Then instruct the patient to move his pupil to the larger [nasal] angle of the eye, looking towards you, similar to looking sidewards to the smaller [temporal] angle of the eye. |

---

21 Literally, this passage translates: "The day should be a northern one and not a southern one and it be a day of sun." It is at first unclear as to what should be a "northern day" or a "southern day." This can be explained, however, after reading Ṣalāḥ ad-Dīn (fragment 5): "On a day where the wind is northern, not southern, and clear of dust." Clearly, in ʿAlī ibn ʿĪsā, the word for wind (al-hawāʾ) got lost, which resulted in a "northern day" and a "southern day" and not in one with northern or southern wind. Judging from the Arabic and considering how the text should be reconstructed, it is evident that both texts refer to the southern and northern wind.

| | |
|---|---|
| keep the distance from the so-called iris to the small corner of the eye, corresponding approximately to the length of the button of the probe; then we press the spot where we want to perform the couching with the button of the cataract needle | Then keep distance from the "wreath" [the iris] to the smaller angle of the eye, according to the size of the tip of the cataract needle. After that, mark the place you want to pierce [in the sclera] with the tail of the cataract needle by pressing on it until there is a kind of indentation in it [the sclera], for two reasons: firstly, so that the patient gets used to being patient and that you test him and, secondly, so that a place is created for the sharp head [of the probe] where it has a firm guidance and where it will not slide away when you want to pierce, lest it should be pushed back. The marking should be opposite the pupil, immediately above, after a very small distance, but not deviating downwards. |
| using the right hand for the left eye and the left one for the right,<br><br>and we turn the tip of the cataract needle, which is rounded at the end, forward by applying constant pressure on it [the cataract needle], through the spot previously indented, until it [the cataract needle] goes into the void [ie, until a sudden decrease of resistance is felt]. | And you should do [the couching] with the left hand if the right eye is concerned and with the right hand if the left eye is concerned. Then turn the cataract needle upside down, place its triangular sharp tip on the spot that you marked before, and forcefully press on it with the cataract needle, until the sclera gets pierced and you notice that the cataract needle entered a wide empty space (*áchri kenembatéseōs* [see fn. 19]). |
| | And if you press on the cataract needle, its sharp tip should be inclined a little to the "small" [= temporal] angle of the eye, because in this way it leaves the remaining layers [of the eye] intact. And [even] if it [the needle] slips out, you are safe. However, before you push in the cataract needle, the thumb and index finger [of your other] hand, which do not hold the cataract needle, should grasp the eyeball from above and from below. And this is done above the eyelids so that the eye does not turn and you are not disturbed by its movement. |

| | |
|---|---|
| A measure for penetrating into the depth is as much as the distance between the pupil and the iris. | And the measure of the part of the cataract needle that penetrates be only as much as reaches to the pupil and does not exceed it. And if it exceeds it by half a barleycorn, it is still permissible. But if it is more than this, it is harmful and abrades [see fragment 5: "scrapes off the color of the uvea"]. And when the cataract needle enters, grasp the patient's head with the fingertips of your hand and place the needle on the lower part of your thumb with which you couched the cataract, like an object that rests. And cheer up the patient with pleasant words in order to calm his fear. But he shall not have eaten anything [before surgery], because [otherwise] vomiting sometimes occurs. And if you notice any of this, let him drink a little of bitter beverages, such as thickened juice of Syrian rhubarb, unripe grapes, and tamarinds. Then put a piece of fresh cotton on the eye and gradually breathe warmly into it. You may decide to suck on it [the eye] as if you drink something, in order to soothe the eye from the irritation. |
| Afterwards, we bring the cataract needle to the top of the cataract— since you can see the bronze [the needle] clearly because of the transparency of the cornea— | Then gradually turn the needle until you see it above the cataract. For the bronze is visible due to the clarity of the cornea layer. However, the layer of the uvea is pushed back at the time of turning the needle, but it is not pierced, because of its sticky surface. And it [the needle] is smooth. And for this reason, the tip of the cataract needle is not sharpened, in order not to injure it [the uvea]. Otherwise, the tip of the cataract needle would be sharpened so that it penetrates faster. After that, have a look where the needle is. If it has not yet reached the location of the cataract, give it a little push. And when it has passed it, pull it back a little until it is just above the cataract. When you have done this, gradually lift the lower part of the cataract needle. |

| | |
|---|---|
| and bring with its [the needle's] help the cataract to the underlying parts. Immediately after it [the cataract] has been couched, we stay a little [with the needle] and do not move it. If the cataract rises again, we couch it downwards once more. | Then the cataract is pressed downwards and the fibrous surface of the uvea attracts it with its rough texture. If after that it [the cataract] descends immediately, wait a little and do not rush to pull out the needle so that it [the cataract] does not rise again and return. And if it rises, push it down a second time. And sometimes the fibrous surface [of the uvea] is sticky and takes the cataract with difficulty. And sometimes the cataract is thin. And there are kinds of cataract, which, when the needle pushes them, descend as if they had fallen into a well. And no trace of them remains whatsoever. And there are kinds of it [the cataract], which descend with difficulty. But if it is tedious and difficult and keeps coming back after you have couched it, then divide it sideways, downwards, upwards, and towards the "smaller" and the "larger" angle of the eye. If it causes trouble, then let the spot bleed, by pushing the needle towards the "smaller" angle of the eye so that a little blood comes out. And mix it [the blood] with the cataract and push it down. Then it will not return. But if in this way an unintended bleeding arises, mix it with the cataract and push it down, for it is safe because it imbues the cataract. And instruct the patient to help you with couching by clearing his throat downwards, from his mouth and not from his nose. Because this helps to couch the cataract. |
| Having couched the cataract, we carefully pull out the cataract needle while turning it. | Once it [the cataract] has descended, gradually pull out the cataract needle by turning it outwards. And the patient whose cataract has been couched has little pain. |

| | |
|---|---|
| Afterwards, we dissolve a little bit of Cappadocian salt in water and instill it [the solution] into the eye. And from outside we apply wool that has been soaked in egg yolk and rose oil and then we bandage; we bandage the healthy eye as well so that [the operated one] is not moved. And we make the patient lie in a subterranean room<br><br>and instruct him not to move at all, | When you have taken out the needle and see that the eye is unharmed, bandage it with egg yolk mixed with rose oil. But whenever you see that there is blood on the spot [of the puncture site], bandage from the outside with crushed salt. Because it [the salt] dissolves it [the blood]. And dress both eyes together with a tight bandage and let the patient sleep on his back in a dark room and support his head from both sides. And instruct him to lie like dead and not to move. |
| | A person should always be with him to serve him. And if he wants something, he should indicate it with his hand. And dress [his] temples with anesthetic substances as a precaution against headaches. And prevent him from coughing, sneezing, talking, and other movements. And when he feels like sneezing, he should rub his nose vigorously, because this way it [the urge to sneeze] decreases. And likewise, if he feels like coughing, he should drink a little of rose water with almond oil; this way it [the urge to cough] ceases. |
| administering him a light diet and keeping him bandaged up to the seventh day if nothing contradicts. | And his food should be light and should not consist of things which are difficult to chew, but [of things] which are fairly easy to eat and which are digested fairly quickly, like vegetables and eggs for slurping. And reduce his food and prevent him from drinking much water. And on the second day completely loosen the bandage, while he sleeps. And gradually remove the bandage, wash the eye with cotton that has been moistened with rose water, and do not touch the eye with it and do not open it. And moisten a piece of cotton with thin egg white, put it on the eye and again dress the whole [both eyes together]. If you do not loosen it [the bandage] until the third day, it is better. And when the third day elapses, loosen it [the bandage] and wash it [the eye] with water in which roses have been boiled. And make him sit down with a pillow behind him against which he leans. |

| | |
|---|---|
| | And he should stay like this, with as little movement as possible. And hang a black rag in front of his face and motivate him until the seventh day. |
| | And if you choose to treat with remedies in the form of a powder, sprinkle hematite or a black collyrium alone, and let it work. And if the cataract rises again during these days [those of the aftercare], then use the needle a second time, unless there is a warm swelling [inflammation], in the same puncture site in his eye, because it does not scar quickly because it is "cartilage." <br><br> And you should know that the conjunctiva is sometimes soft and the cataract needle does not penetrate it. Then first use a scalpel that has a round tip and insert the cataract needle after that. And beware of a plethora [of humors] in the [patient's] body or of him having a headache. Because it destroys what you are doing. I have repeated these words for the sake of safety. And sometimes excess flesh is generated in the site you have pierced. Do not be afraid of it, take it away with the tip of a pair of scissors, and it will heal ... |

**Fragment 4 on Cataract: Commentary**

Fragment 4 is from the *Memorandum for Ophthalmologists* by 'Alī ibn 'Īsā (ca. 940-1010 AD). In chapters II.73-74 of this treatise, the etiology, symptomatology, and therapy of cataracts are extensively discussed and described. Antyllus is nowhere quoted or mentioned by 'Alī ibn 'Īsā, either in these chapters or elsewhere. However, 'Alī ibn 'Īsā's cataract chapter not only has the same framework and content as Paul's chapter, but many surplus passages, some of which occur verbatim in fragments 1, 2, and 3, here expressly labeled by Rāzī as being from Antyllus, but not preserved in Paul's Greek. It is, therefore, evident that 'Alī ibn 'Īsā made extensive use of an Arabic Antyllus translation, not only in the cataract chapter but also in the other chapters that have the same peculiarities and links to Antyllus. In principle, one could view all of 'Alī ibn 'Īsā's chapters II.73-74 as Antyllus fragments. However, there would be need to prove this by an external source with overlapping content and clear author indication. The duplicate passages in Rāzī only double validate short sections. More such passages would be needed to validate Antyllus' authorship for the rest. In addition, it can be assumed that 'Alī ibn 'Īsā edited the text extensively, incorporating his own observations and comments as well as passages from other unnamed authors. Hirschberg and Lippert (1904), who translated the entire 'Alī ibn 'Īsā, indicate parallels to Paul in footnotes. Since this type of presentation makes a systematic comparison impossible, a synoptic form of comparison is chosen here. For fragment 4, only those passages (with the associated context) from chapters II.73-74 were chosen that can be double validated by fragments 1-3 with their author indication "Antyllus."

**Fragment 5 on Cataract: Translation**

| Translation from the Greek of Paul of Aegina 6.21 (ed. Heiberg 1921-1924 [CMG]) | Translation from the Arabic of Ṣalāḥ ad-Dīn, p. 422.2seqq. (ed. al-Wafā'ī, 1987) |
|---|---|
| (2.) … We make the patient sit facing the light, but not in direct sunlight; | How to couch a cataract: If one wants to couch a cataract, the patient must sit in the shade, in a place where his face is opposite the sunshine, on a day when the wind comes from the north, not from the south, and when it is free from dust. And there should not be food in his [the patient's] stomach so that he does not vomit. And let him drink a drink of Syrian rhubarb, unripe grapes, peppermint, and tamarind. It should best be done at the time of the equinoxes, in spring, and in autumn. And the patient should sit on a soft padding and bring his knees to his chest; and bring his hands together on his thighs. Sit on a chair so that you are positioned higher than him. |
| we carefully bandage the healthy eye, | And bandage his healthy eye very tightly with a compress. This is because there are two benefits: The first is that the eye does not move at the time of healing and the other one consequently does not move either. Otherwise you would not be able to do your job. The other benefit is if the cataract has successfully been couched and you let the patient whose cataract has been couched see something, one does not say that he [the patient] sees with his healthy eye. And instruct a person [an assistant] to stand behind him and to hold his head. Then he [the assistant] should lift the upper eyelid [of the patient] in order to expose to you the whole eye. Then place your thumb firmly, coming from above, to fix the eye. And instruct the patient to look at the left inner angle of the eye, towards the nose, similar to looking sideways. And keep that position. |
| spread the lids of the other one, | |

| | |
|---|---|
| (a) then we press the spot where we want to perform the couching with the button of the cataract needle, (b) | Then press [the sclera] with the [blunt] tail of the cataract needle, until a pit is created on it, at a distance from the cornea equal to the length of the tip of the cataract needle, so that the patient gets used to having patience and that the sharp tip of the cataract needle has a place from which it does not slip away. |
| keep the distance from the so-called iris to the small corner of the eye, corresponding approximately to the length of the button of the probe; (a-b) -> (c) | **Antyllus:** The distance of the cataract needle from the pupil should be according to the distance of the pupil from the margin of the pupil. And the [blunt] mark should be at the margin of the pupil, just above, after a very small distance, so that the cataract needle acts on the cataract when it encounters it. |
| (e) and we turn the tip of the cataract needle, which is rounded at the end, forward by applying constant pressure on it [the cataract needle], through the spot previously indented, (f)<br><br>(c) using the right hand for the left eye and the left one for the right, (d)<br><br>(g) until it [the cataract needle] goes into the void [ie, until a sudden decrease of resistance is felt]. | Then press firmly on the marked spot, with the sharp triangular tip of the cataract needle,<br><br><br><br>if it is the right eye, with the left hand, and if it is the left eye, with the right hand, until the conjunctiva is pierced and you feel that the cataract needle enters the void [*áchri kenembatéseōs*, see fn. 19]. |
| A measure for penetrating into the depth is as much as the distance between the pupil and the iris. | And the length of the cataract needle that enters corresponds to the pupil. And if it exceeds the length of half a barleycorn, this is permissible. More than this, however, scrapes away the coloring of the uvea. The sharp tip of the cataract needle should be slightly inclined towards the "small" [temporal] angle of the eye, because this leaves the remaining layers intact. And when the cataract needle enters, hold the patient's head with your hand and push the needle on the lower part of your thumb, which you used to couch the cataract, so that he [the patient] calms down. Then cheer him [the patient] up with pleasant talk and soothe his fear [this way]. |

| | |
|---|---|
| (h) Having couched the cataract, we carefully pull out the cataract needle while turning it. (i) Afterwards, we bring the cataract needle to the top of the cataract … and bring with its [the needle's] help the cataract to the underlying parts. (h-i) | Then put freshly sheared cotton on the eye and breathe warmly into it. If you decide to suck on it [the eye] as if you drink something, in order to soothe the eye from the irritation, then gradually turn the needle until you see it behind the corneal layer. At the time of turning the needle, the uvea is pushed back, but not pierced because of the stickiness on it. Then gradually lift up the lower part of the cataract needle, for the cataract will be pressed downwards [this way]. The stickiness of the uvea attracts it. |

## Fragment 5 on Cataract: Commentary

Fragment 5 is a passage from the treatise *Light of the Eyes* by the Arabic ophthalmologist Ṣalāḥ ad-Dīn. The treatise was written around 1296 AD.[22] In contrast to fragment 4, fragment 5 only corresponds to the second section of Paul's cataract chapter, with numerous textual expansions. In contrast to fragment 4, fragment 5 is not transmitted anonymously, since the author indication "Antyllus" can be found in the second half of the fragment. For reasons of consistency in content and due to textual parallels to fragment 4, Antyllus' authorship must also be assumed for the first section of fragment 5.

A total of four descriptions of the cataract operation, which go back to Antyllus, have been preserved in Arabic. These four descriptions have, however, a different scope, show different levels of detail in various items, and sometimes also have a different order of arguments.

When comparing these four descriptions, one first notices a particular closeness between Ṣalāḥ ad-Dīn and ʿAlī ibn ʿĪsā, which emerges not only in terms of content but also through the many literal similarities between both authors. However, the text in Ṣalāḥ ad-Dīn appears to be somewhat rearranged compared to ʿAlī ibn ʿĪsā. Since Ṣalāḥ ad-Dīn is the chronologically later author, who gives a shorter text than ʿAlī ibn ʿĪsā and since there are no passages that do not also appear in ʿAlī ibn ʿĪsā (who is mentioned elsewhere in Ṣalāḥ ad-Dīn's text by name[23]), one may conclude that Ṣalāḥ ad-Dīn excerpted from ʿAlī ibn ʿĪsā.

---

22   See Hirschberg/Lippert/Mittwoch p. 198.
23   See Hirschberg/Lippert/Mittwoch p. 199.

## Fragment 6 on Cataract: Translation

> ### Translation from the Arabic of 'Alī ibn 'Īsā (p. 264.3-11 ed. Khan, 1964)
>
> And forbid him [the patient to do] cupping and [to eat] thick foodstuffs, especially those that moisten such as beef, sheep fat, broad beans, cheese, milk, dates, and lentils; [forbid him to] drink wine, especially the young one, [forbid him] constant bathing, sexual intercourse, fasting, eating vegetables such as onions, leeks, basil, and anything similar to these. And especially forbid him to eat fish. Because it is one of the things that cause the formation of cataracts. ... And he should only eat at lunchtime.

## Fragment 7 on Cataract: Translation

> ### Translation from the Arabic of Ṣalāḥ ad-Dīn, p. 411.10seqq. (ed. al-Wafā'ī, 1987)
>
> **Antyllus:** He who suffers from cataract should avoid cupping, eating fish and sheep meat, wine, and legumes. And he should eat [only] once, in the middle of the day.

## Fragments 6 and 7 on Cataract: Commentary

The hypothesis that Ṣalāḥ ad-Dīn excerpted from 'Alī ibn 'Īsā seems to be confirmed by another pair of fragments (fragment 6/7): Fragment 7, from Ṣalāḥ ad-Dīn, describes dietary measures for cataract patients under the name of Antyllus. It particularly deals with which foodstuffs they should avoid. A very similar, but much more detailed passage can be found in 'Alī ibn 'Īsā (fragment 5). One may assume that fragment 7 is a summary of this text passage, which can be identified as an Antyllus passage through fragment 7. It seems apparent once more that Ṣalāḥ ad-Dīn excerpted from 'Alī ibn 'Īsā. The problem, however, is that, in both cases, Ṣalāḥ ad-Dīn has the author indication "Antyllus" in his text, which is nowhere mentioned in 'Alī ibn 'Īsā.

Accordingly, it cannot be ruled out that both authors go back to a third (unknown) source that contained Antyllus' name or that both authors independently drew from a complete Arabic translation of Antyllus' surgical manual. Ṣalāḥ ad-Dīn—despite using 'Alī ibn 'Īsā—could also have added the name "Antyllus" in both instances, maybe because he recognized, by comparison with other sources, that 'Alī ibn 'Īsā drew from Antyllus. But given the fact that fragment 7 is very short and that it deals with less relevant subjects, this explanation seems less probable.

A comparison of the Antyllus fragments 1 and 2, which are preserved in Rāzī's *Ḥāwī*, with the ones from 'Alī ibn 'Īsā and Ṣalāḥ ad-Dīn (fragments 4 and 5) shows that the latter two fragments have a lot of excess text. It is not clear whether this surplus goes back to Antyllus or whether it was supplemented by 'Alī ibn 'Īsā (or his source). Based on the current state of research and the sources known so far, this question cannot be answered. Only by finding further passages, which, like fragment 7, contain the author reference "Antyllus," further passages from 'Alī ibn 'Īsā could be identified as Antyllus fragments.

## Fragment 8 on Cataract: Translation

**Translation from the Arabic of Rāzī, Ḥāwī (I 79vII Par. = 41vII Ven. (book 2.3) = II.202.4 Haid.)**

**Antyllus says:** And [some] people cut at the lower border of the pupil and remove the cataract. **He says:** And this is only done in the smooth cataract, not in the hard one, because the egg-like moisture [= aqueous and/or vitreous humor] flows out together with that [form of] cataract. And [some] people insert a glass tube into the place of the drilling hole [of the cataract needle] and suck on it [the cataract]. Together with it [the cataract], they suck out the egg-like moisture.

## Fragment 9 on Cataract: Translation

**Translation from the Arabic of Ṣalāḥ ad-Dīn, p. 429.19seqq. (ed. al-Wafā'ī, 1987)**

**Rāzī, second book of Ḥāwī, from Antyllus:** Some people incise at the lower part of the pupil and remove the cataract. And this is what happens in the thin cataract. But not in the thick one, because the egg-like fluid flows together with this cataract. And there are people who insert a glass tube into the place of the drilling and suck. They suck out the egg-like fluid together with it [the cataract]. And among the views that support 'Amār's view are the words of Antyllus concerning the incision of the lower part of the pupil, although this is very dangerous for the cornea and although the scar develops at the place of the separation of continuity; and because of the proximity [of the incision] to the egg-like [fluid], it flows [out].

## Fragment 10 on Cataract: Translation

**Translation from the Arabic of Ḥalīfa, p. 314.15-17 (ed. al-Wafā'ī, 1987)**

**In his memorandum book, Manṣūr mentions that the Greek ophthalmologist says:** I saw some people incising the lower part of the pupil and extracting the cataract. And this is what happens with the smooth cataract. But not with the hard one, because the egg-like moisture flows out together with this [kind of] cataract.

## Fragment 11 on Cataract: Translation

**Translation from the Arabic of Ḥalīfa, p. 318.6seq. (ed. al-Wafā'ī, 1987)**

**Manṣūr says in his memorandum book:** I saw people inserting a glass tube into the site of the cataract needle and sucking out the egg-like moisture together with the cataract.

**Fragments 8-11 on Cataract: Commentary**

The remaining fragments (8-11) deal with two alternative methods of cataract treatment, by making an incision at the lower edge of the pupil and sucking out the cataract with a glass tube. Unfortunately, these fragments are extremely brief. They only mention the procedure, but not how exactly it is performed. The method of cataract extraction by cutting is also attested by Galen during Greco-Roman antiquity.[24] Fragments 8-10 emphasize that cataract extraction after cutting is only possible with a thin cataract, since, in a thick one, the "egg-like moisture" (ie, aqueous and/or vitreous humor of the eye) would flow out with the cataract. In fragment 8 from Rāzī's Ḥāwī (also in fragment 9, which refers to this passage in Rāzī), the suction method is mentioned after the cutting method, introduced by the remark "and [sc. some] people ..." It is questionable whether Antyllus is still quoted here or whether this second part (the comment on the suction method) derives from another author. Fragment 9 is from Ṣalāḥ ad-Dīn. Herein, he simply quotes Rāzī's passage from fragment 8 (with the cutting and sucking method) and then mentions Antyllus, with reference to the cutting method. Fragment 10, from Ḥalīfa's ophthalmological treatise (to be dated around 1256 AD[25]), quotes a certain Manṣūr, who, in turn, quotes "the Greek ophthalmologist," Antyllus. Only the cutting method is mentioned here. In fragment 11, Ḥalīfa quotes Manṣūr again, concerning the cutting method. The suction method is mentioned once more, in comparable wording to the other passages, but only under the name of Manṣūr, not of Antyllus.

No source explicitly mentions the suction method under Antyllus' name. In all of the second book of Rāzī's Ḥāwī, which deals with ophthalmology, Julius Hirschberg compared the quotations from Greek authors in Rāzī with the Greek original. He found out that, in many instances in Rāzī's Ḥāwī, an addition is made to the quotations from the Greeks. Without comparing the original sources, these additions could not have been recognized as such.[26] Considering this and the fact that the suction method is always introduced with "some people" (once as an appendix to an Antyllus quotation [fragment 8] and once alone under the name Manṣūr [fragment 11]), Hirschberg suggests that this is an interpolation from an Arabic source (Hirschberg et al., 1905). Therefore, the suction method should not be associated with Antyllus and not be viewed as an Antyllus fragment. Nevertheless, Meyerhof (1933, p. 78) continues to do so. As for the cutting method, there are no doubts of this kind, since it is always quoted with the author indication "Antyllus."

---

24  See Galen Methodus medendi 14,13 (X,987,11-13 Kühn), Meyerhof (1933) p. 73. and Feugère et al. (1985), pp. 486-488.

25  See Hirschberg/Lippert/Mittwoch p. 155.

26  See Hirschberg (1904), p. 226 and Hirschberg (1905), p. 231seq.

# References and Abbreviations

## Abbreviations

CMG = *Corpus Medicorum Graecorum* series.

CML = *Corpus Medicorum Latinorum* series.

Haid. = Osmania University (ed.) (1955-71).

Par. = *Codex Parisinus Latinus* 6912.

Ven. = Faragut (translator), O. Scoto (publisher): *Continens Rasis ...*, Venice 1529.

## Text Editions, Translations

Adams F. The Seven Books of Paulus Aegineta. Translated from the Greek with a Commentary. London: Sydenham Society; 1844-47.

Berendes J, Paulos von Aegina. *Des besten Arztes sieben Bücher*. Übersetzt und mit Erläuterungen versehen. Leiden: 1914.

*Codex Parisinus Latinus* 6912. Available online from: https://archivesetmanuscrits.bnf.fr/ark:/12148/cc90779w [References to this work are abbreviated "Par." in this chapter].[27]

Faragut (trans.), Scoto O (publisher). Continens Rasis ... liber quem in medicina edidit Abuchare filius Zacharie Rasis ... Hunc Helchauy, hoc est Continentem appellavit ..., Venice: O Scoto; 1529. [References to this work are abbreviated "Ven." in this chapter].[28]

Heiberg JL (ed.). Paulus Aegineta, pars prior: libri I-IV, pars altera: libri V-VII. Leipzig/Berlin; 1921-1924 (CMG IX,1-IX,2).

Hirschberg J, Lippert J, Mittwoch E. *'Ammār b. 'Alī al-Mauṣilī, Das Buch der Auswahl von den Augenkrankheiten, Ḫalīfa al-Ḥalabī, Das Buch vom Genügenden in der Augenheilkunde, Ṣalāḥ ad-Dīn, Licht der Augen, aus arabischen Handschriften übersetzt und erläutert*. Leipzig: 1905.

Khan, 'Abdul-Muʿīd (ed.). *'Alī ibn 'Isā al-Kaḥḥāl, Taḏkirat al-kaḥḥālīn*. Hyderabad; 1964.

Kühn KG. *Claudii Galeni Opera Omnia*. 20 vols. Leipzig: 1821-1833 (reprint: Hildesheim: 1997).

Marx F (ed.). *A. Cornelii Celsi quae supersunt*. Leipzig/Berlin; 1915 (reprint: Hildesheim: 2002) (Corpus medicorum Latinorum [CML] 1).

Olivieri A (ed.). *Aetii Amideni Libri medicinales*, libri i-iv, libri v-viii. Leipzig/Berlin; 1935-1950 (Corpus medicorum Graecorum [CMG] VIII,1-VIII,2).

Osmania University (ed.). *Abū Bakr Muḥammad ibn Zakarīyā ar-Rāzī, Kitāb al-Ḥāwī fī ṭ-ṭibb*, 23 vol., Hyderabad/Deccan: Osmania University; 1955-71. [References to this work are abbreviated "Haid." in this chapter].[29]

Scheller E, Frieboes W. *Aulus Cornelius Celsus: Über die Arzneiwissenschaft in acht Büchern*. Mit einem Vorworte von [...] R Kobert, Braunschweig; 1906 (reprint: Hildesheim: 1967).

al-Wafā'ī, Muḥammad Ẓāfir (ed.). *Ṣalāḥ ad-Dīn, Nūr al-ʿuyūn, Ṣalāḥ-ad-Dīn Ibn-Yūsuf al-Kaḥḥāl al-Ḥamawī, Nūr al-ʿuyūn wa-ǧāmiʿ al-funūn*. ar-Riyāḍ; 1987.

---

27 References to this manuscript have the format "I 79vII Par.," which means: first volume of this manuscript, folium 79 verso, column 2. For folium 79 recto, column 1 the reference would be I 79rI.

28 References to this edition have the format "41vII Ven. (book 2.3)," this means: folium 41 verso, column 2; "book 2.3" added in brackets means book 2, chapter 3 of the Latin translation, which is often different from the book and chapter count of the edited Arabic text.

29 References to this edition have the format II.202.4., which means: volume 2, page 202, line 4. If the line is counted backwards from the bottom of the page, this is indicated by a minus sign, for example, II.202.-4.

## Secondary Literature

Allen WS. Vox Graeca. *A Guide to the Pronunciation of Classical Greek*. Cambridge; 1987.

Feugère M, Künzl E, Weisser U. Die Starnadeln von Montbellet (Saône-et-Loire). *Ein Beitrag zur antiken und islamischen Augenheilkunde / Les aiguilles à cataracte de Montbellet (Saône-et-Loire)*. Contribution à l'étude de l'ophthalmologie antique et islamique, in: Jahrbuch des Römisch-Germanischen Zentralmuseums Mainz, 1985: 436-508.

Fischer K-D. Die Klappe fällt—frühe Belege für lat. cataracta als Bezeichnung einer Augenkrankheit. *Medizinhistorisches Journal* 2000;35(2):127-147.

Fischer K-D. Ὄνπερ τρόπον οἱ ἰατροὶ ἐν ἀνθρώπῳ, in: Müller CW, Brockmann C, Brunschön CW (ed.), Ärzte und ihre Interpreten, Medizinische Fachtexte der Antike als Forschungsgegenstand der Klassischen Philologie, Fachkonferenz zu Ehren von Diethard Nickel. München/Leipzig; 2006: 203-224.

Grant RL. Antyllus and his Medical Works, in: *Bulletin of the History of Medicine* 1960;34:154-174.

Hirschberg J. Die Instrumente der arabischen Augenärzte, in: *Centralblatt für praktische Augenheilkunde* 1904;28:161-173.

Hirschberg J. Die Staroperation nach Antyllos, in: *Centralblatt für praktische Augenheilkunde* 1906;28:97-100.

Hirschberg J. *Geschichte der Augenheilkunde*. Berlin: Registerband; 1918.

Hirschberg J. Lippert J. *Ali ibn Isa, Erinnerungsbuch für Augenärzte, aus arabischen Handschriften übersetzt und erläutert*. Leipzig; 1904.

Ihm S. *Clavis commentariorum der antiken medizinischen Texte*. Leiden etc.; 2002.

Kalbfleisch K. *Simplicii in Aristotelis categorias commentarium*. Berlin; 1907 (Commentaria in Aristotelem Graeca 8).

Magnus H. *Die Augenheilkunde der Alten*. Breslau; 1901.

Meyerhof M. L'opération de la cataracte du chirurgien Antylle d'Alexandrie (IIième siècle après J-C), in: Koumaris J, Rosenauer F, Sackarndt B (ed.), *Livre d'or à l'occasion du jubilé de vingt-cinq ans d'activité chirurgicale du docteur Théodore L. Papayoannou*. Kairo/Naumburg; 1932: 115-119.

Meyerhof M. Die Operation des Stars in der griechischen Medizin, in: *Die Antike, Zeitschrift für Kunst und Kultur des klassischen Altertums* 1933;9:72-80.

Pansier P. *Collectio Ophthalmologica Veterum Auctorum*, vol. 2. Paris; 1903.

Weisser U. Die Rezeption der Methodus medendi im Continens des Rhazes, in: Kudlien F, Durling RJ (eds.), *Galen's Method of Healing*. Leiden etc.; 1991: 123-146.

Wellmann M. Antyllos 3, in: *Paulys Realencyclopädie der classischen Altertumswissenschaft*, vol. I,2. Stuttgart; 1894: 2644-2645.

Wellmann M. *Die pneumatische Schule bis auf Archigenes*. Berlin; 1895.

Witt M. (forthcoming-a). Die chirurgische Operationslehre (Χειρουργούμενα) des Antyllos von Alexandrien (2. Jh. n. Chr.)—eine kommentierte Rekonstruktion und medizinhistorische Analyse anhand der überlieferten griechischen und arabischen Fragmente, Habilitation thesis University of Munich (LMU), forthcoming in the *Studies of Ancient Medicine series*, Leiden etc.

Witt M. (forthcoming-b). Zur Frage der wechselseitigen textuellen Abhängigkeit der spätalexandrinischen Chirurgiehandbücher (des Leonides, Archigenes, Heliodoros und Antyllos), aufgezeigt an den Kapiteln über den Wasserkopf und an weiteren Textstellen, forthcoming in *Sudhoffs Archiv*.

# A *New History of Cataract Surgery* consists of:



* Chapters origination from: *The History of Ophthalmology – The Monographs 15: The History of Glaucoma*